MW01233249

<u>WEIGHT LOSS HYPNOSIS</u>

2 IN 1 BOOKS, STOP EMOTIONAL EATING & SUGAR CRAVINGS AWAKENING MOTIVATION AND SELF ESTEEM. FOR WOMEN AND MEN THAT WANT TO BURN FAT QUICKLY WITH GASTRIC BAND HYPNOSIS RISK FREE

RAPID WEIGHT LOSS HYPNOSIS:

LOSE WEIGHT NATURALLY THROUGH SELF-HYPNOSIS AND AFFIRMATIONS TO INCREASE SELF-ESTEEM AND MOTIVATION. BURN FAT QUICKLY WITH NATURAL GASTRIC BAND, HEALING YOUR BODY & SOUL.

Introduction 7

Chapter 1 Understanding Hypnosis 15

Chapter 2 What Exactly is Hypnosis? 32

Chapter 3 Hypnosis and the Power of Mind 40

Chapter 4 Hypnosis and Weight Loss 48

Chapter 5 Re-Program Your Mind 55

Chapter 6 Self-Hypnosis Session 61

Chapter 7 The Great Power of Meditation 69

Chapter 8 Guided Meditation 77

Chapter 9 Affirmations and Subconscious Mind.................. 84

Chapter 10 Positive Affirmation for Weight Loss 92

Chapter 11 Repetition Like a Mantra 99

Chapter 12 Sharp Your Mind to Shape Your Body..............106

Chapter 13 Heal Your Relationship with Food 114

Chapter 14 We Shall Talk Here About Breakfast in Order to Really Know Why It Is So Important. 115

Chapter 15 Mindful Eating Habits... 122

Chapter 16 How to Practice Every Day............................... 126

Chapter 17 Self-Love 132

Chapter 18 Stop Emotional Eating 140

Chapter 19 Portion Control Hypnosis 148

Chapter 20 Additional Tips to Help You Lose Weight.........154

Chapter 21 Overcoming Negative Habits 161

Chapter 22 Mistakes to Avoid... 168

Chapter 23 The Importance of Habits.................................172

Chapter 24 Frequently Asked Questions 177

Chapter 25 Create Reasonable Goals.................................. 185

Chapter 26 Learn to Avoid Temptations and Triggers........ 192

Chapter 27 How to Build Motivation................................... 199

Chapter 28 Strategies and Mind Exercises..........................203

Conclusion... 211

GASTRIC BAND HYPNOSIS FOR WEIGHT LOSS:

Sharpen your mind to shape your body. rapid weight loss self-hypnosis to Stop Food Addiction, burn fat quickly and Eat Healthy, with Permanent Results.

Introduction 219

Chapter 1: Self – Hypnosis 225

Chapter 2: What is Hypnosis? 230

Chapter 3: Positive Self Talk vs. Negative Self Talk............ 239

CHAPTER 4: Subconscious Mind 244

Chapter 5: The Power of Visualization.......................252

Chapter 6: Meditation to Release Stress.................... 261

Chapter 7: Hypnosis and Meditation 267

Chapter 8: What is a Gastric Band? 276

Chapter 9: Strong Hypnotic Gastric Band - The Weekly Program. 284

Chapter 10: Healing Yourself – Relaxation Techniques.......291

Chapter 11: Maintaining a Strong Daily Practice 300

Chapter 12: Believe 306

Chapter 13: All-natural Ways to Burn Fats.....................314

Chapter 14: The Four Golden Rules 321

Chapter 15: Tips and Tricks 329

Chapter 16: Living a Healthy Habit Life............................... 335

Chapter 17: Discover the Satisfaction Factor 343

Chapter 18: Motivational Affirmations 349

Chapter 19: Gain Confidence 356

Chapter 20: Fall in Love with Your Body 363

Chapter 21: Positive Impacts of Affirmations 367

Chapter 22: Tips to Help You Succeed with No Stress 375

Chapter 23: Enjoy the Experience of Nurturing and Taking Care of Your Body...382

Chapter 24: Eat Healthy and Sleep Better with Hypnosis... 391

Chapter 25: The Psychology about Weight Loss 399

Chapter 26: Women are Different from Men........................406

Chapter 27: Blasting Calories 411

Chapter 28: Great Techniques to Reach Your Ideal Weight 420

Conclusion...428

RAPID WEIGHT LOSS HYPNOSIS:

LOSE WEIGHT NATURALLY THROUGH SELF-HYPNOSIS AND AFFIRMATIONS TO INCREASE SELF-ESTEEM AND MOTIVATION. BURN FAT QUICKLY WITH NATURAL GASTRIC BAND, HEALING YOUR BODY & SOUL.

Introduction

While brainwashing is a notable type of mind control that numerous individuals have about, hypnosis is additionally a significant sort that ought to be thought of. Generally, the individuals who know about hypnosis think about it from watching stage shows of members doing silly acts. While this is a sort of hypnosis, there is much more to it. This part is going to focus more on hypnosis as a type of mind control.

What is Hypnosis?

To begin with, what is the meaning of hypnosis? As indicated by specialists, hypnosis is viewed as a condition of cognizance that includes the engaged consideration alongside thdiminished fringe mindfulness that is described by the member's expanded ability to react to recommendations that are given. This implies the member will enter an alternate perspective and will be substantially more defenseless to following the recommendations that are provided by the trance inducer.

It is broadly perceived that two hypothesis bunches help to depict what's going on during the hypnosis time frame. The first is the changing state hypothesis. The individuals who follow this hypothesis see that hypnosis resembles a daze or a perspective that is adjusted where the member will see that their mindfulness is, to some degree, not quite the same as what they would see in their normal cognizant state. The other hypothesis is non-state speculations. The individuals who follow this hypothesis don't believe that the individuals who experience hypnosis are going into various conditions of awareness. Or maybe, the member is working with the subliminal specialist to enter a sort of inventive job authorization.

While in hypnosis, the member is thought to have more fixation and center that couples together with another capacity to focus on a particular memory or thought strongly. During this procedure, the member is likewise ready to shut out different sources that may be diverting to them. The mesmerizing subjects are considered to demonstrate an increased capacity to react to recommendations that are given to them, mainly when these proposals originate from the subliminal specialist. The procedure that is utilized to put the member into hypnosis is knitted hypnotic enlistment and will include a progression of suggestions and guidelines that are used as a kind of warm-up.

There is a wide range of musings that are raised by specialists with regards to what the meaning of hypnosis is. The wide assortment of these definitions originates from the way that there are simply such huge numbers of various conditions that accompany hypnosis, and nobody individual has a similar encounter when they are experiencing it.

Some various perspectives and articulations have been made about hypnosis. A few people accept that hypnosis is genuine and are suspicious that the legislature and others around them will attempt to control their minds. Others don't have faith in hypnosis at all and feel that it is only skillful deception. No doubt, the possibility of hypnosis as mind control falls someplace in the center.

There are three phases of hypnosis that are perceived by the mental network. These three phases incorporate acceptance, recommendation, and defenselessness. Every one of them is critical to the hypnosis procedure and will be talked about further underneath.

Induction

The principal phase of hypnosis is induction. Before the member experiences the full hypnosis, they will be acquainted with the hypnotic enlistment method. For a long time, this was believed to be the strategy used to place the subject into their hypnotic stupor. However, that definition has changed some in current occasions. A portion of the non-state scholars has seen this stage somewhat in an unexpected way. Instead they consider this to be as the strategy to elevate the

Members' desires for what will occur, characterizing the job that they will play, standing out enough to be noticed to center the correct way, and any of the different advances that are required to lead the member into the proper heading for hypnosis.

There are a few induction procedures that can be utilized during hypnosis. The most notable and compelling strategies are Braid's "eye obsession" method or "Braidism." There are many varieties of this methodology, including the Stanford Hypnotic Susceptibility

Scale (SHSS). This scale is the most utilized instrument to examine in the field of hypnosis.

To utilize the Braid enlistment procedures, you should follow several means. The first is to take any object that you can find that is brilliant, for example, a watch case, and hold it between the centers, fore, and thumb fingers on the left hand. You will need to hold this item around 8-15 crawls from the eyes of the member. Hold the item someplace over the brow, so it creates a ton of strain on the eyelids and eyes during the procedure with the goal that the member can keep up a fixed gaze on the article consistently.

The trance inducer should then disclose to the member that they should focus their eyes consistently on the article. The patient will likewise need to concentrate their mind on that specific item. They ought not to be permitted to consider different things or let their brains and eyes meander or, in all likelihood, the procedure won't be effective.

A little while later, the member's eyes will start to enlarge. With somewhat more time, the member will begin to accept a wavy movement. If the member automatically shuts their eyelids when the center and forefingers of the correct hand are conveyed from the eyes to the item, at that point, they are in the stupor. If not, at that point, the member should start once more; make a point to tell the member that they are to permit their eyes to close once the fingers are conveyed in a comparable movement back towards the eyes once more. This will get the patient to go into the adjusted perspective that is knaps hypnosis.

While Braid remained by his method, he acknowledged that utilizing the acceptance procedure of hypnosis isn't always fundamental for each case. Analysts in current occasions have typically discovered that the acceptance strategy isn't as essential with the impacts of hypnotic recommendation as recently suspected. After some time, different other options and varieties of the first hypnotic acceptance procedure have been created, even though the Braid strategy is as yet thought about the best.

Recommendation

Present-day sleep induction utilizes a variety of proposal shapes to be fruitful, for example, representations, implications, roundabout or non-verbal recommendations, direct verbal proposals, and different metaphors and recommendations that are non-verbal. A portion of the non-verbal suggestions that might be utilized during the recommendation stage would incorporate physical manipulation, voice tonality, and mental symbolism.

One of the qualifications that are made in the kinds of recommendation that can be offered to the member incorporates those proposals that are conveyed with consent and those that progressively tyrant in the way.

Something that must be considered concerning hypnosis is the contrast between the oblivious and the cognizant mind. There are a few trance specialists who see the phase of the proposal as a method of conveying that is guided generally to the conscious mind of the subject. Others in the field will see it the other way; they see the correspondence happening between the operator and the subconscious or oblivious mind.

They accepted that the recommendations were being tended to directly to the conscious piece of the subject's mind, as opposed to the oblivious part. Braid goes further and characterizes the demonstration of trance induction as the engaged consideration upon the proposal or the predominant thought. The fear of a great many people that subliminal specialists will have the option to get into their oblivious and cause them to do and think things outside their ability to control is inconceivable as per the individuals who follow this line of reasoning.

The idea of the mind has additionally been the determinant of the various originations about the recommendation. The individuals who accepted that the reactions given are through the oblivious mind, for example, on account of Milton Erickson, raise the instances of utilizing aberrant recommendations. Huge numbers of these aberrant proposals, for example, stories or representations, will shroud their expected importance to cover it from the cognizant mind of the subject. The subconscious recommendation is a type of hypnosis that depends on the hypothesis of the oblivious mind. If the unconscious mind were not being utilized in hypnosis, this sort of recommendation would not be conceivable. The contrasts between the two gatherings are genuinely simple to perceive; the individuals who accept that the recommendations will go fundamentally to the cognizant mind will utilize direct verbal guidelines and proposals while the individuals who accept the proposals will go essentially to the oblivious mind will use stories and analogies with concealed implications.

This permits them to be driven toward the path that is required to go into the hypnotic state. When the recommendation stage has been finished effectively, the member will, at that point, have the option to move into the third stage, powerlessness.

Powerlessness

After some time, it has been seen that individuals will respond contrastingly to hypnosis. A few people find that they can fall into a hypnotic stupor reasonably effectively and don't need to invest a lot of energy into the procedure by any means. Others may find that they can get into the hypnotic daze, however, simply after a drawn-out timeframe and with some exertion. Still, others will find that they can't get into the hypnotic stupor, and significantly after proceeding with endeavors, won't arrive at their objectives. One thing that specialists have discovered intriguing about the weakness of various members is that this factor stays steady. If you have had the option to get into a hypnotic perspective effectively, you are probably going to be a similar path for an incredible remainder. Then again, if you have consistently experienced issues in arriving at the hypnotic state and have never been entranced, at that point, almost certainly, you never will.

There have been a few distinct models created after some time to attempt to decide the defenselessness of members to hypnosis. A portion of the more established profundity scales attempted to construe which level of a daze the member was in through the discernible signs that were accessible. These would incorporate things, for example, the unconstrained amnesia. A portion of the more present-day scales works to quantify the level of self-assessed or watched responsiveness to the particular recommendation tests that are given, for example, the immediate proposals of unbending arm nature.

As per the examination that has been finished by Deirdre Barrett, there are two kinds of subjects that are considered profoundly vulnerable to the impacts of subliminal therapy. These two gatherings incorporate dissociates and fantasizers. The fantasizers will score high on the assimilation scales, will have the option to effortlessly shut out the boosts of this present reality without the utilization of hypnosis, invest a great deal of their energy wandering off in fantasy land, had fanciful companions when they were a youngster, and experienced childhood in a situation where nonexistent play was energized.

Chapter 1
Understanding Hypnosis

Hypnosis in Psychology

Whereas NLP is a pseudo-science, hypnosis and hypnotherapy have been accepted by the medical establishment as viable methods of behavior modification and therapeutic psychological treatment. Hypnosis is also referred to as hypnotherapy or hypnotic suggestion.

According to the Mayo Clinic, hypnosis is defined as "a trance-like state in which you have heightened focus and concentration...usually done with the help of a therapist using verbal repetition and mental images."

The word hypnosis is derived from the Greek word "hypnos," which means "sleep." There is some debate about who first developed the theory and practice of hypnosis. Many people believe hypnosis was first developed in the 19th century. Some people credit the French researcher Étienne Félix d'Henin de Cuvillers who had spent time trying to understand how people in a deep state of relaxation would respond to suggestions to change their behavior. Others have credited James Braid, a Scottish surgeon who has been given credit for first calling the practice "hypnosis."

Many of the humorous and negative stereotypes of hypnosis can be credited to 18th century German physician Franz Mesmer. Mesmer conducted many experiments and demonstrations in his efforts to prove what he referred to as "animal magnetism." He believed an invisible fluid flowed between living animals, people, and plants, and that by influencing the direction and rate at which this fluid flowed, he could create behavioral changes. His attempts to prove this so-called "animal magnetism" were eventually discredited, and his practices were shown to be dishonest and lacking in any scientific validity. However, his earlier efforts eventually led to further research. In addition, his influence has been long-lived—we still refer to excellent artistic performances or engrossing dialog as "mesmerizing."

Contemporary hypnotherapy consists of two functions: Induction and suggestion. During hypnotic induction, the therapist attempts to place the patient into a deep state of relaxation. Once the patient has achieved a hypnotic state, the therapist makes suggestions designed to help the patient achieve the desired behavior. The following diagram illustrates the degree to which we are influenced by our subconscious mind, the reason so many people turn to hypnotherapy to help them change deep-seated behavior:

Myths about Hypnosis

Dispelling the many stereotypes of hypnosis is the first step in understanding this area of psychotherapy. The sideshow practitioner with a big moustache who dangles or spins a large object with a spiral design in front of the patient until they fall under his spell occurs only in movies.

• **Myth #1**—Patients cannot remember what happens during hypnosis.

It is not true that patients under hypnosis cannot remember anything when they are pulled back out of the hypnotic state. Patients under hypnosis are generally fully aware of everything during hypnosis and remember everything that occurs during a session.

In some cases, as when a hypnotherapist suggests to the patient that he or she forgets certain things that occurred immediately before or during a session, the patient may experience posthypnotic amnesia, but this effect may result from a deliberate effort to help the patient recover from a psychological difficulty, and in most cases it is limited and temporary. Amnesia has been reported in some cases, but it is infrequent.

•**Myth #2**—Hypnosis can help patients remember forgotten events.

Television crime shows often portray the power of psychics and hypnotherapists to solve crimes by helping traumatized victims recall details from the crime scene that allow lawyers and police officers to crack the case, but the idea that hypnosis can help patients retrieve forgotten details or memories of past events has been largely disproven.

There is some evidence that hypnosis can help improve memory overall. However, studies have shown that in instances in which hypnosis has been used to help patients retrieve lost memories or achieve so-called "past life regression," the results were more likely false memories or fictitious recollections resulting from suggestions during the trance state.

•**Myth #3**—Hypnotherapists can put you under a spell and make you do anything.

It is a myth that anyone can be hypnotized against their will or forced to act in ways that violate their beliefs or morality. In order for hypnosis to be effective, the patient must be a willing and active participant. Similarly, when the patient is fully hypnotized, the hypnotist does not have complete control over the actions of the patient under hypnosis. People who are hypnotized may be less inhibited to act in specific ways, but even in a trance state, patients are not able to work in ways they believe are wrong or that violate their morals or ethics.

•**Myth #4**—Hypnosis can give patients superhuman abilities.

Popular culture sometimes portrays the limitless possibilities that can open up to patients who undergo hypnosis. Film and television may portray hypnotherapy sessions in which the patient is convinced that when he or she comes out of the trance state, they will be able to run faster than a car, be smarter than anyone else at work, lift automobiles, or resist bullets. Hypnotherapy can help patients improve their performance in a variety of areas—both physical and mental. But it cannot allow anyone to exceed the limits of their own physical or intellectual abilities.

Facts about Hypnosis

In actual practice, hypnotherapy is much less dramatic and exciting than the portrayals in popular film and television. In fact, many people enter a hypnotic state every day. A hypnotic state is defined as a very relaxed and focused psychological state in which the subject is very calm, focused, susceptible to suggestion, and less likely to be influenced by hesitations or inhibitions.

For example, every time you sit down at home or in a movie theater to watch a film, you enter a hypnotic state. As the movie begins, your mind shifts its attention from concerns about work, family, relationships, bills, and other daily concerns to the story that is about to unfold. Especially if the lights are dimmed and outside interference from sounds and activity is muffled or blocked, your mind gradually relaxes and begins to shift its focus more and more to the film, until at some point you are entirely engrossed by the images, sounds, and events on the screen. Often during these episodes, we enter such a deep state of hypnosis that we react to scenes of violence, comedy, or shock as if they were actually happening.

In professional environments, many contemporary work gurus have developed the idea of "flow." When you are at work and so focused on what you are doing that it ceases to require any strain or effort, you have entered a state of "flow." When you are in this state, you are capable of producing high quality work that may generally seem excessively tricky. What's more, you may be able to sustain this high level of productivity for hours on end and even derive an intense sense of pleasure and happiness. This, too, is a state of hypnosis.

Hypnosis is usually used in combination with psychotherapy. During psychotherapy, patients may have explored many of the painful or difficult thoughts or feelings they have been experiencing. Under hypnosis, they may be more willing to explore these areas in more depth, which can lead to a better resolution.

What Are the Uses of Hypnosis?

Patients under hypnosis feel calm and relaxed and are generally more open to suggestions. The main uses of hypnosis are for resolving problems associated with physical illnesses, behavioral problems, and psychological ailments.

•**Physical conditions:** Hypnotherapy can help patients who are having difficulty with any of the following physical illnesses:

Chronic or Acute Pain

Many patients who have been diagnosed with rheumatoid arthritis or post-surgical pain have benefited from hypnotherapy by altering the patients' perception of pain. In one experiment, a patient under hypnosis was instructed not to feel any pain in his arm. The patient then placed his arm in a tub of icy ice water and was able to leave it therefore several minutes without experiencing any pain. Patients in the same experiment who had not been hypnotized had to remove their arms from the water after only a few seconds.

Pain Associated With Medical Procedures

Patients who are undergoing dental care, childbirth, or other painful medical procedures have benefited from undergoing hypnotherapy prior to treatment.

Migraine headaches

Because migraine headaches are often triggered by stressful conditions, hypnotherapy can help reduce their frequency and intensity without the side effects of medication.

Irritable Bowel Syndrome (IBS)

This condition can cause considerable discomfort. Although not effective as a long-term treatment on its own, hypnotherapy can help patients resolve short-term discomfort associated with IBS.

Side Effects From Cancer Treatment

Chemotherapy to treat certain forms of cancer can cause considerable discomfort and nausea. Hypnotherapy has been effective in helping some patients alleviate these side effects.

Skin conditions, including warts, psoriasis, and eczema

Some skin conditions can be triggered by stress and anxiety. In these cases, helping patients find a way to resolve chronic anxiety can help relieve symptoms.

•**Behavioral changes:** Hypnosis can also be used to effect behavioral changes, such as in treatments for the following conditions:

Insomnia

Patients who have insomnia may also be suffering from stress-related conditions. Hypnotherapy can help patients learn new habits and techniques to help the patient fall asleep without medication.

Smoking, Overeating, Bed-Wetting

Addictions and other behavioral problems can be difficult to resolve using only therapy and medication. Hypnosis can help patients learn to change their behavior in areas where they have been resistant.

•Emotional and psychological disorders: Finally, hypnotherapy is sometimes used to treat the mental health problems listed below.

Stress and anxiety

Stress and anxiety disorders are often treated with medication. However, such treatment may only address symptoms and may result in harmful side effects. Hypnosis can provide an additional source of relief for patients suffering from this condition.

Phobias

Phobias are a challenging and complex area of psychology. Though there is no single answer for why someone may have developed a particular fear, hypnotherapy can help the patient change his or her perceptions and reactions to triggers.

Post-traumatic Stress Disorder

Also known as PTSD, this condition is similar to stress and anxiety disorders but usually caused by an acute or sudden traumatic experience. The effects can cause long-term problems and hypnotherapy can help patients find healthier ways of responding.

Grief and Loss

Grief and loss can lead to ongoing challenges for many people. By helping patients refocus their attention, hypnotherapy can aid in a quicker recovery.

Depression

There are many causes of depression. Sometimes patients have been in difficult circumstances, while others may be psychologically predisposed to depression, Often, it is a combination of factors. Regardless, hypnosis can help patients redirect their mental focus and find relief.

Dementia

Patients with dementia may have trouble concentrating and remembering. Hypnosis has been shown to be effective at helping them reconnect with familiar surroundings.

Attention Deficit and Hyperactivity Disorder (ADHD)

The growing concerns about this psychological ailment have resulted from the quickened and disjointed pace of work and life in environments that use digital technology. Hypnosis can help patients adjust to a less stressful setting and develop a longer attention span.

Self-Hypnosis

The only significant difference between hypnosis and self-hypnosis is that in the first one, the operator and the subject are two different people. In self-hypnosis, the operator and the issue coincide in the same person.

It is also a fact that learning is more comfortable and faster when done with another person.

Ask your partner to hypnotize you using a procedure similar to the one we used in the second session. Then practice the self-hypnosis exercise for a few days. Ask your partner once again to hypnotize you and reinforce hypnotic suggestion. Practice it again.

The number of times it is necessary to reinforce the procedure depends entirely on you. If you practice the daily self-hypnosis exercise, one or two reinforcement sessions will be sufficient.

But what about those who have no one with whom to share the learning experience of self-hypnosis? What can they do?. How can they learn?

Leave your worries aside.

It is possible to use self-hypnosis to solve virtually any type of problem and broaden your consciousness and connect with your innate superior intelligence and creative ability. By using self-hypnosis for the latter purpose, hypnosis can transform into meditation.

Self-hypnosis can also be used in those moments when you feel the need for a higher power to intervene in some situations; Then, it becomes a prayer. The subtle differences between these forms of self-hypnosis lie in the way thoughts guided once the state of consciousness itself has altered, that is when the alpha state has reached.

Then I will tell you a fun experience that happened to me with self-hypnosis. I had an appointment with the dentist to have two molars removed. Last night I had conditioned myself to stop the flow of blood.

On the day of the appointment, when sitting in the dentist's chair, I self-reported. When the dentist removed the teeth, I blocked the flow of blood so that it did not flow through the open wound. The dentist was perplexed and kept telling his assistant: «It doesn't bleed.

How is it possible?. I don't understand it. I smiled since I couldn't physically smile because of all the devices, cotton, and objects that held my mouth. Besides, I visualized quick and complete healing. After seventy-two hours the swelling had subsided, and the wounds had healed completely;

And now, I will tell you another funny experience that one of my patients had with self-hypnosis.

He was part of a group that participated in an investigation about dreams at the local hospital. Once a week, my patient slept in the hospital with an electroencephalogram (EEG) connected to his head. This was intended to record the waves of their brain activity.

By observing the graph, doctors could establish if they were an alpha, beta, tit, or delta, and they could also state when the patient was sleeping and when he was awake. My client immediately hypnotized himself as soon as he connected to the EEG.

The apparatus recorded a deep alpha state, indicative that the subject was sleeping, although he was fully awake. One of the doctors asked: "What's going on here?" Then the man alternately returned to the beta state, then to alpha, then again to beta, and finally to alpha while the machine registered it.

The changes confused the doctors until the subject told them what he was doing. The response of the doctors cannot reproduce here.

I have devised and written practically all the contents of this guidebook in an alpha state. What does this mean?. It means that it is possible to develop an activity and keep your eyes open even if one is in an altered state of consciousness. Think about it for a moment.

It transports us to another state while we are comfortably and quietly sitting with our eyes closed, thinking about a specific objective. But using self-hypnosis in this sense is not easy to achieve since it requires a prolonged period of preconditioning in a hypnotic or autohypnotic state. Such preconditioning is similar to that used for diet control, but the indications are different; It will be necessary to devise the techniques and suggestions for this case.

And it also requires practice, a lot of practice. Do not forget my words; time and effort will reward with the results. Develop your discipline and stick to it; The results will be a real success.

Hypnosis Step by Step Procedure

1. Believe. A significant part of the intensity of spellbinding lies in your conviction that you have a method for assuming responsibility for your desires. If you don't figure entrancing will enable you to change your emotions, it will probably have little impact.

2. Become agreeable. Go to a spot where you may not be stressed. This can resemble your bed, a couch, or a pleasant, comfortable chair anyplace. Ensure you bolster your head and neck. Wear loose garments and ensure the temperature is set at an agreeable level. It might be simpler to unwind if you play some delicate music while mesmerizing yourself, particularly something instrumental.

3. Focus on an item. Discover something to take a gander at and focus on in the room, ideally something somewhat above you. Utilize your concentration for clearing your leader of all contemplations on this item. Make this article the main thing that you know about.

4. Breathing is crucial. When you close your eyes, inhale profoundly. Reveal to yourself the greatness of your eyelids and

let them fall delicately. Inhale profoundly with an ordinary mood as your eyes close. Concentrate on your breathing, enabling it to assume control over your whole personality, much like the item you've been taking a gander at previously. Feel progressively loose with each fresh breath. Envision that your muscles disperse all the pressure and stress. Permit this inclination from your face, your chest, your arms, lastly, your legs to descend your body. When you're entirely loose, your psyche should be clear, and you will be a self-mesmerizing piece.

5. Display a pendulum. Customarily, the development of a pendulum moving to and from has been utilized to energize the center is spellbinding. Picture this pendulum in your psyche, moving to and from. Concentrate on it as you unwind to help clear your brain.

6. Start by focusing on 10 to 1 in your mind. You advise yourself as you check down that you are steadily getting further into entrancing. State, "10, I'm alleviating. 9, I get increasingly loose. 8. I can feel my body spreading unwinding. 7, Nothing yet unwinding I can feel.... 1, I'm resting profoundly. Keep in mind that you will be in a condition of spellbinding when you accomplish 1 all through.

7. Waking up from self-hypnosis. Once during spellbinding, you have accomplished what you need, you should wake up. From 1 to 10, check back. State in your mind: "1, I wake up. 2, I'll feel like I woke up from a significant rest when I tally down. 3, I think wakeful more.... 10, I'm wakeful, I'm new.

8. Develop a plan. Reinventing your mind with spellbinding requires consistent redundancy. You ought to endeavor in a condition of spellbinding to go through around twenty minutes per day. While beneath, shift back and forth between portions of the underneath referenced methodologies. Attempt to assault your poor eating rehearses from any edge.

9. Learn to refrain from emotional overeating. One of the main things you should endeavor to do under mesmerizing is to influence yourself. You are not intrigued by the frightful nibble of food you experience issues kicking. Pick something that you will, in general, revel in like frozen yogurt. State "Dessert tastes poor and makes me feel debilitated." Repeat twenty minutes until you're prepared to wake up from the trance. Keep in mind; excellent eating regimen doesn't suggest you have to quit eating, simply eat less awful sustenance. Simply influence yourself to devour less food, you know, is undesirable.

10. Write your very own positive mantra. Self-spellbinding ought to likewise be utilized to reinforce your longing to eat better. Compose a mantra to rehash in a trance state. It harms me and my body when I overeat.

11. Imagine the best thing for you. Picture what you might want to be more beneficial to support your longing to live better. From when you were slenderer, take a picture of yourself or do your most extreme to figure what you'd resemble in the wake of shedding pounds. Concentrate on this image under mesmerizing. Envision the trust you'd feel on the off chance that you'd be more advantageous. This will cause you to comprehend

that when you wake up. Eat each supper with protein. Protein is especially valuable at topping you off and can improve your digestion since it advances muscle improvement. Fish, lean meat, eggs, yogurt, nuts, and beans are great wellsprings of protein. A steak each dinner might be counterproductive, yet in case you're eager, eating on nuts could go far to helping you accomplish your objectives.

12. Eat a few, modest meals daily. If you don't eat for quite a while, your digestion will go down, and you will stop fat consuming. If you expend something modest once every three or four hours, your metabolism will go up, and when you plunk down for dinner, you will be less hungry.

13. Eat organically grown foods. You will be loaded up with foods grown from the ground and furnish you with supplements without putting any pounds on. To start shedding pounds, nibble on bananas rather than treats to quicken weight reduction.

14. Cut down on unhealthy fats. It tends to be helpful for you to have unsaturated fats, similar to those in olive oil. Nonetheless, you should endeavor to limit your saturated fat and trans-fat intake. Both of these are significant factors that add to coronary illness.

15. Learn more about healthy cooking. In preparing meals, trans fats are common, mainly when eating meals, sweets, and fast food.

16. Saturated fats may not be as bad as trans fats. However, they might be undesirable. Primary saturated fat sources include spreads, cheddar cheese, grease, red meat, and milk. The journey to weight loss is not an easy one. A person needs a lot of help and motivation to succeed. With the help of hypnotherapy, one can

easily stay the course and watch the pounds melt away. Following the guide above and with a credible hypnotherapist or mastering self-hypnosis will help you achieve your goals.

Chapter 2
What Exactly is Hypnosis?

History

Hypnotism has been around since ancient times and in fact, the entire concept and development of hypnotherapy and hypnosis can be found in old documents and texts. Hypnosis was in practice for several centuries but gained massive popularity only in the 18th century. It is believed that the French were the first to develop and fine-tune hypnosis and make it into a practicing art form. In the 1840s James Braid was the one who coined the term hypnotism. In this technique, he believed that hypnosis was more of a self-centered approach and awareness rather than just mesmerizing somebody. There are several texts and documents that throw the significance of hypnosis. While many believed that the French were the original founders, there are several scripts from forgotten eras, which prove otherwise.

According to several historians like Will Durant, he didn't believe that the French founded hypnotism. He thought that the Indians used hypnotism as a tool. He believed that the Hindus found in India were the first to practice hypnotism extensively. Gurus, Rishis, and other hermits practiced the art of meditation, concentration, and focus. This was believed to be done to communicate with the Hindu gods and goddesses. Also, people who fell sick in ancient India were taken to monks who sat and meditated at temples. These monks cured the problems and ailments of the people who came to them through hypnosis. Other sources claim that Avicenna from Persia distinguished between hypnotic trance and sleep. This Persian psychologist stated the differences in his book 'The Book of Healing'. In his book, he says that hypnosis is a state in which a person can induce conditions and situations to one person and the other person can accept this as reality.

There has also been wide speculation about magnetism and mesmerism in hypnotism. It is also believed that hypnotism was developed through these two. For instance, Valentine Greatrakes from Ireland became popular due to his ability to use magnets and heal his patients. He was termed as "the Great Irish Stroker" due to his talent. Paracelsus was a physician from Switzerland who used magnets to treat people, which were proved to be very useful. A Catholic priest called Johann Joseph Gassner healed people through hypnotism. He advocated that those diseases that were caused by evil spirits would leave the body through meditation and prayer. In the 17th century, Father Maximilian Hell who was a Jesuit from Vienna used magnets by placing them on the body of the patients to heal them. One of his apprentices was Franz Anton Mesmer, who developed modern forms of hypnosis.

Franz Anton Mesmer was an Austrian physicist, who revolutionized hypnosis. He researched and developed something known as mesmerism, which is alternatively known as animal magnetism. In this form, he distinguished between traditional magnetism that was done with the use of magnets and animal magnetism that referred to the force that each person possessed inside them. Human beings and animals could exercise this force in order to enhance themselves. Inspirited by the works of Richard Mead who was an English physician, Franz Anton Mesmer discovered that after a patient bled, they were able to develop resistance by using a magnet and passing it over the cut. The magnetic force made the bleeding stop. He gained massive popularity in France especially with the rich and influential citizens of France for his ability to cure people using magnets. It was at this point that the medical community faced stiff competition from him and hence put forth a challenge. Heeding to the request of the medical community, the French aristocrats and kings formulated a board consisting of a chemist called Lavoisier, a medical doctor whose expertise lied in controlling pain called Joseph Ignace Guillotin and Benjamin Franklin. Mesmer refused to participate in this challenge and declined to answer any questions that the board put forward. He instead made his apprentice Dr. D'Eslon who experimented on a patient. He blindfolded the patient and the results showed the responsiveness of the patient in comparison to that of a tree, which has been magnetized. The board accepted this and believed that mesmerism could be put into practice only by using the imagination. Though, this form of therapy is an alternate form that has gained massive popularity, Mesmer kept to himself and retired to Switzerland where he subsequently died.

With Mesmer's coinage came a lot of support. There were several advocated of this style of practice. During the French revolution, mesmerism was used to control the crowd. In fact, ancient texts and records give detailed description on how the French aristocrats brought together people who practiced this art. There are suggestions made stating that social order could be restored through mesmerism. It was at that period that magnetism started to wear off. People stopped using magnetism extensively and switched to mesmerism. Abbé Faria was an Indo Portuguese priest who channeled the interest of the public into animal magnetism. He formulated what the Parisians knew as oriental hypnosis in the 19th century. He hailed from India and traveled across the world and exhibited his style of magnetism. He did not make use of patients nor did he confirm to medical reasons. He also did not manipulate to achieve results. The major difference between the mesmerism style developed by Mesmer and Faria's oriental hypnosis was that Faria believed that the forces were developed from the mind of the person. Through cooperation and training, people could project themselves a lot better and enhance their minds. His style of hypnosis was researched upon, extended and case studied by practitioners like Hippolyte Bernheim and Ambroise-Auguste Liébeault. The framework that Faria had developed and the extension and fine-tuning of Faria's theories by several people contributed to the development of new techniques like the autogenic training techniques which were developed by Johannes Heinrich Schultz and the autosuggestion techniques which were founded by Émile Coué. Marquis de Puységur was the first to introduce the term somnambulism. He was an apprentice of Mesmer and his followers and disciples were called

Experimentalists. They were advocated of the theory of Paracelsus Mesmer fluids.

Like stated before the exact founding of hypnotism is unknown and there are several texts from the 18th century. One of these is those of Récamier who used a particular form of hypnotism before its actual founding and popularity. He was a physician who used a type of hypnotism that was similar to hypnoanesthesia where he cured his patients after lulling them into a mesmeric coma. After him, Carl Reichenbach researched extensively on this energy that Récamier used. Though several believed that Récamier possessed magical and supernatural powers, Carl Reichenbach tried to find a scientific explanation to this energy. This energy was termed after the Norse god Odin and was called Odic force. The scientific community that existed rejected all of Reichenbach's arguments and explanations. It was in 1846, after the publishing of the literary work called 'The Power of the Mind over the Body' by James Braid that Reichenbach's explanation was termed as pseudoscientific.

However, extensive use of hypnotism in some form or the other spread. This was exclusive to the 18th century alone. In fact, the mesmeric sleep technique was used as an anesthetic in British occupied India. Physician James Esdaile operated upon about 350 people by lulling them into a state of conscious coma through mesmeric practices. This was used before the advent of chemical anesthetic. This practice was significantly reduced after synthetic anesthetic was discovered. Hypnosis was still used in certain inaccessible pockets of the world. A surgeon called John Elliotson from England also carried this out. He used hypnosis to perform operations. These operations proved to be successful and painless due to the use of hypnosis.

How Hypnosis Works

Hypnosis is not what many people think it is. Because of old movies and performers, many people tend to believe that hypnosis is some form of party trick that results in people struggling to have any control over themselves and their behaviors. This is actually not at all true. When you are engaging in hypnosis, you always remain in control of yourself, your body, and your behaviors. The suggestions being offered to you in guided meditations are just that: suggestions. Because hypnosis is not the absolute power that many movies depict it as it can take a few tries with hypnosis before you get the results you are looking for out of it. Many people will use about 3-4 sessions per area of focus in order to start seeing significant results. Some people may use up to 8-10 sessions before they experience absolute resolve of the issue that leads them to seek out the power of hypnosis in the first place.

When you are engaged in a hypnosis session, you are mainly relaxing to the point where you can sink deeper into your awareness. Think of this as being similar to dreaming without actually being asleep. Through this deep state of relaxation and the ability to sink into your more in-depth awareness, you are able to take suggestions from guided meditations and permanently rewire your subconscious mind. A great example of this is when people use self-hypnosis as a way to encourage themselves to increase their self-esteem. In this case, they are introducing positive thoughts about self-esteem and self-confidence into their subconscious minds so that they can begin to have a new mental experience around the topic of themselves.

As you "awaken" into your subconscious mind and introduce these new thoughts, you give your brain the opportunity to change how it works completely. Now, rather than your subconscious mind feeding your conscious mind unhelpful thoughts and perspectives, your subconscious mind will feed your conscious mind, helpful ideas, and different perspectives that support your preferred reality. For example, with your self-esteem, this could result in you having thoughts that reinforce your self-confidence and a reality that fosters a more profound sense of self-esteem.

When it comes to your weight loss goals, your primary focus is on changing your subconscious mind around food. This way, you can eliminate any habits or behaviors that lead to compulsive eating, cravings, or overeating, and you can begin to instill new habits and practices on a subconscious level. What ends up happening is that when you awaken into your reality, you notice that you no longer have such intense cravings or urges around food, and you are able to have more pleasant and positive experiences with your diet.

Creating these changes on a subconscious level means that you are able to have an entirely renewed perspective around food and weight loss. Now, rather than depriving yourself, growing frustrated with cravings, or feeling defeated by your diets, you can feel confident and in alignment with your changes. Instead of having to fight off urges within yourself, you simply will not have them to begin with. This may seem too right to be true, but once you start to engage in hypnosis and experience the changes in your subconscious mind, you will see just how powerful hypnosis actually is.

Chapter 3

Hypnosis and the Power of Mind

Subconscious Mind (Unconscious Mind)

This is the portion of our psyche performing functions and processes below our awareness of thinking. It is the body's mind. It breathes us, digests us, beats our hearts and controls our unconscious physical processes for us in general. It can also tell us to pick a slice of fresh fruit instead of a chocolate cake, avoid eating when we're full or take a walk through the park.

Entering Trance

When you're using the audio trance job, I'll be your guide as you get into trance. I'll use a form of trance induction that you will find relaxing and concentrating. You probably saw the swinging watch method in movies, which I have never seen anybody use in thirty-five years of practice, but there are many different ways to focus your attention on going into trance. You may stare at a wall spot, use a breathing technique, or use progressive relaxation of your body. On the trance job recording you'll hear a variety of induction's methods. These are simply the signs or signals you send yourself to say "I 'm going into trance" or "I 'm going to do my hypnosis now." Going into trance can also be thought of as "letting yourself daydream ... intentionally." You're letting yourself be immersed in your thoughts and ideas, really distracted, and enabling yourself to think or visualize what you want to do and what you want to accomplish. There is no "going under." Instead there is a lovely feeling of going inside.

The Trance Deepens

Deepening your trance helps you absorb your thoughts, ideas and experience more. This is achieved with incremental relaxation: moving "deeper and deeper within ..." of photos or scenes, for example, or counting a sequence of numbers. We like to suggest that you create a vertical image associated with going more in-depth, such as a path leading down a mountain or into a lush green valley, as you hear the counting from ten down to null. You can visualise or imagine going deeper into a scene or location that's even more fun and relaxing for you as you hear me count. We mean this with "deepening the trance."

Conscious Mind

This is the "conscious mind" or part of the psyche that gives us a sense of intelligence or consciousness and regulates our voluntary functions. For instance, our conscious mind at the buffet takes that second piece of pie, swipes the debit card at the grocery store, and moves the fork to our mouth.

Talking to the Mind of Your Body with Messages and Suggestions

During the trance work, you will hear my voice speaking to two parts of your mind. One part of your mind is your conscious thinking mind, which is the part of you that is great at telling time, making change, learning how to read and write; it is your "thinking mind." Throughout the trance phase, your thinking mind will continue doing its normal activity of having thoughts. So, you don't have to think about clearing your mind, or emptying your mind, or setting your mind totally at peace. Simply notice that your mind will start "thinking," and your task is to unplug or isolate just enough so that you do not have to respond to those thoughts. You give them permission to stream by. If your "to do" list keeps popping up, for example, just allow it to stream by, rather than dwell on it.

The other part of your mind I will be speaking to is what we call your subconscious mind— "sub" because it is below your thinking level of awareness. It is the "mind of your body." Your subconscious mind has the wisdom to manage your body's trillions of cells, your body chemistry, and all the body's functions of breathing, digestion, the nervous system, the endocrine system, and the immune system. The mind-body contains an immense amount of wisdom, and, in doing your hypnosis, you are accumulating and acquiring additional knowledge that the mind of your body will act upon, consistent with your motivation, your beliefs, and your expectations, to help you with your weight loss as well.

You always have the opportunity to adjust and tailor the words being spoken or the images described to best fit you. This tailoring process is crucial. It has to fit you, because it is your self-hypnosis, and all hypnosis is self-hypnosis. As we've said, hypnosis is not something done to you. It is something that you are being guided to experience, and by doing so, you are learning it. Repetition and rehearsal build in your solid ability and knowledge. You may even term its subconscious awareness, because your subconscious mind can do it for you without also having to think about it. So, the thoughts and ideas that might have bothered you about your weight, or your weight loss failure, are now being turned into something that embraces your perfect body. And your mind-body memorizes the experience so that rather than the unwanted results of the past, it can refer to that experience.

For example, if you think you're a "yo-yo" dietitian because you've always recovered the weight you've lost, you may use your trance work to say, "I lose weight every day, and my body knows how to make this a permanent capacity. I 'm able to get my perfect weight. "Subconscious awareness, or mind-body experience gained from your trance work, is much like learning to ride a bike or drive a car. When you first discovered, there seemed to be a lot of things to pay attention to at the same time, but your mind-body took on this information really fast so you can drive safely now, and there is no need to tell your feet what to do.

One of our clients, Amy, told us that she would tell her body what she wanted her ideal weight to be, when she first began using self-hypnosis. In the set-point of body weight, she would dial carefully and vividly, with a picture of changing a thermostat to the number of pounds she desired. She'd focused on these images. Her mind-body has replied with a few imaginative tests. She found out that her weight fluctuated around the set-point she imagined within just one plus-or minus-five-pound range. As if she would automatically experience a craving for fruits and vegetables as her weight increased, and forget about desserts. She also felt more inclined to exercise, and felt full before she finished a meal. She described the results: "To make these changes automatically for me now is like my body has an autopilot."

Getting Out of Trance

At the end of the trance work sessions, you'll hear me talking about letting your body wake up with a feeling of refreshment and well-being, and bringing that refreshment with you to the front surface of your mind so that you'll be comfortably renewed and alert from the trance feeling. Or you might be slipping into a deep, restful sleep when you do your hypnosis at bedtime.

It is important to debrief after you are on the alert. If thoughts or ideas came to mind that would be useful to you, this is the time to make a note or two for yourself. Often during the trance, you're not just sending your body instructions, but your body is talking to you and you'll listen to your body's mind. You can share beneficial information with your body and you might want to write it down.

Let's say, for example, that you have a particular food you just can't resist, a food like French fries that was your "downfall" in dieting. You can get an insight during the trance-work (something you learned when you listened to your body's mind) that tells you why French fries emotionally are an obstacle to you, or even a "comfort." The knowledge now allows you to choose what you want and not merely implement the earlier pattern that was formed, maybe decades ago, and born out of some emotional experience that is now long past and no longer true in your life.

Jennifer was diligent and hardworking in every area of her life and almost every aspect of her weight loss program. Every day she exercised, ate plenty of fruits and vegetables, drank plenty of tea, enjoyed grains and even bought organically whenever she could. She made very wise health choices, but stayed 20 pounds over her perfect weight. When she sat in our office miserably, she told every night about her almost insatiable appetite for ice cream (organic though it was) and any social opportunity that presented itself. We asked during her trance-work if there was a part of her that understood why she seemed to be craving ice cream. She was quiet for several minutes and then repeated her caring grandfather's long-ago words: "Jenny, darling, ice cream is the greatest reward for hard work, so eat up while you have the chance to, maybe it's gone tomorrow, just like me." Once she realized the root of her ice cream addiction, she might enjoy it but not eat it too much.

Hypnotic Phenomena

Trance is an exceptionally subtle experience. You should study the subtleties of what you have heard, what you have not seen and what you have encountered. Some people may feel heavy, almost immovable in their arms and legs; or they may feel lighter, weightless or floating. Some may feel warm or cold, or become so lost in the mental imagery that they feel as if they are in fact there, present in their imagination. Parts of the body may seem so totally gone that they're not even seen. It's also typical that time be experienced differently. One minute might sound like ten minutes, or ten minutes might just seem like one. These are natural events that we call "hypnotic phenomena." If you are familiar with daydreaming, you should also know that the majority of what is considered hypnotic phenomena are also common wake-state phenomena. How many times have you been "awakened" from a daydream, or roused from an exciting book or film, to find that a surprising amount of time has passed?

There is a broad variety of potential symptoms with hypnosis, including hypnoanalgesia (the pain reduction) and hypnoanesthesgia (the pain elimination). A person can possibly imagine, when in trance, that a part or more of her body is so comfortably numb that she can undergo surgery using hypnosis as the sole aesthetic.

You will be pleased to know that hypnotic phenomena which are particularly useful for weight loss can be produced. For example, you might be able to create a physical feeling of fullness, or a desire for nourishing food. You may create a sensation of enhanced taste or odour. You might even be able to forget foods that don't match your weight loss targets. You may also be surprised to feel a craving for exercise.

Remember that self-hypnosis is strong. You can choose what you want your mind-body to say. You can pick what you wish your mind-body to do for you. It's your decision, your weight to make.

Chapter 4
Hypnosis and Weight Loss

Hypnosis for losing weight is a therapeutic hypnosis (hypnotherapy), called Ericksonian. It should not be confused with "spectacle" hypnosis during which the practitioner takes control of his subject. Focused on relaxation, hypnosis for weight loss is a very different approach. During the session, you remain conscious and entirely in control of yourself. The hypnotherapist is there to guide you gently and help you better understand where the eating behaviors that cause your weight gain come from. By this serene journey to the heart of your subconscious, you profoundly modify specific conditioning and lousy eating habits.

Alternative medicine par excellence, hypnosis for losing weight is a powerful tool that will allow you to (re) take control and regain your ideal weight durably and without frustration.

Lasting Weight Loss With Hypnosis

Of course, losing weight necessarily involves questioning one's eating habits. Since we have to go through this, it is legitimate to wonder how hypnosis for losing weight concretely triggers these changes in perception. During the session, the therapist immerses his patient in a profound state of relaxation. His goal encourage him to access his subconscious mind and specific automatisms / conditioning which are the cause of his bad eating habits. Accompanied by the voice of the hypnotherapist, the patient deconstructs his relationship to food. This is, for example, to suggest to his subconscious that high calorie foods are not the only ones that do him right.

This deep introspective work is the guarantee of lasting weight loss. Losing weight through hypnosis therefore meets the expectations of those who seek to lose weight permanently ... without going through the frustration box!

Effectiveness of Hypnosis Session For Losing Weight

What to expect

The idea of losing weight with hypnosis arouses your curiosity? Because we all have the spectacular spectacle hypnosis in mind, we very often associate this practice with a total loss of control.

Provided by a qualified hypnotherapist, a hypnosis session to lose weight lasts 1 hour and leaves you entirely free to move and think. First stage? An essential exchange that will allow your practitioner to identify your problem and personalize this hypnosis session to lose weight.

With relaxation techniques, your therapist guides you to a deep state of letting go. This hypnotic state, known as a second and modified state, will then allow you to gain gentle access to your unconscious and to the conditioning responsible for your weight gain.

If the voice and the expertise of the practitioner accompany you throughout the session, it is you who walk in the heart of your subconscious and are the actor of these profound inner changes.

More and more people recognize the benefits of hypnosis to help people lose weight and maintain a healthy and stable weight over time. Beyond simple testimonials, there are scientific studies that prove the effectiveness of hypnotherapy. One of the first studies on this subject, conducted in 1986, showed that overweight women who used a hypnosis program lost significantly more weight (about 8 kg) than those who were simply told to be careful what they ate. Another study showed that women who used hypnosis to lose weight had slimmed down, improved their body mass index, changed their eating behaviors and even developed a more positive body image.

In the accompaniment of weight loss, the hypnotherapist is a kind of coach, who will first of all help his patient to enter a state of deep relaxation. Once this state is acquired, the hypnotherapist will be able to access the patient's subconscious, which is more open to suggestions than the conscious part of the mind. The hypnotherapist seeks to break the bad eating habits of the patient by replacing the patterns of thought that lead to overeating with more positive and balanced attitudes in relation to food, through visualizations and suggestions.

Thus, hypnotherapy is an approach to weight loss that is based on a change in the relationship with food in the long term: it is to change the way of thinking of the patient, so that these thoughts are translated in healthier actions vis-à-vis its diet. Hypnotherapy is therefore not for those who are looking for "miracle" solutions: it is a process that is undoubtedly effective, but takes time. Changing a patient's attitude towards food requires a good knowledge of the particular problems of the food, and the development of suggestions that respond precisely to his problems. Thus, the first step in any hypnosis for weight loss is going to be a conversation between the therapist and his patient, so that the latter explains his history in terms of diets, what has helped or complicated his weight loss before, etc. Thus, any person thinking of hypnosis as a weight loss technique must abandon the express attitude that accompanies many diets: it is a therapy aimed at a total change in lifestyle and behavior towards feed screw.

Thus, thanks to the power of suggestion, the hypnotherapist can replace negative thoughts and unhealthy behaviors by redirecting them towards actions better for the health of the individual: the hypnotherapist will in no case propose a diet, but helps to adopt a new way of life. Hypnosis allows people to deal with psychological problems that can explain lousy lifestyle habits, such as hatred of sports, excessive greediness, binge eating, etc. It is used to identify the psychological concerns that trigger these bad habits, in order to correct them and create more positive patterns. So one of the critical aspects of hypnotherapy's work in weight loss is going to be to convince the patient that he can lose weight, and that these past failures do not affect the possibility of present success. A big problem with people trying to lose weight repeatedly is that they think their bad habits are "stronger" than they are: the hypnotherapist helps chase away those negative thoughts.

In connection with this, behavioral and cognitive therapy, which is done with the accompaniment of a mental health professional, can be an excellent complement to hypnotherapy: this type of psychotherapy allows the patient to talk about feelings and thoughts that he has in relation to food, which will enable him to be fully aware of the thought patterns and problems at the source of his unhealthy relationship with his diet: subsequently, it will be easier for him to change their habits. Indeed, being aware of the problem is the first step towards more appropriate practices. Another advantage of hypnotherapy in relation to weight loss is that it can also help individuals to manage their stress better: thus, faced with difficult everyday situations, the individual learns to control his emotions in a healthy way. Consequently, he breaks the link between his emotional life and food, which takes up an appropriate place in his existence: it is the way to satisfy his hunger, and not a method to drown his negative emotions in the face of distressing situations. In addition, the meditation and relaxation aspects necessary for hypnosis help the individual to be more aware of his feelings, whether it be his thoughts or his physical state: this can also help to lose weight.

Using Hypnosis to Overcome the Mental Barriers

We create habit patterns through repetition, and with time, they become automatic responses to the environment.

Deep in our minds, we have strong ideas that keep us thinking of unhealthy behaviors. Over time, people train the mind to believe that unhealthy behaviors, as in the case of emotional eating or overindulging, are necessary to maintain our well-being. And as such, if the mind repeatedly thinks of these behaviors, long-term changes become very difficult.

Emotional eating is just an example of associations that negatively affect our efforts to lose weight. There are several other associations that people develop, which impact their relationship with food negatively. Some of these associations that hinder weight loss include:

- Food and constant eating help in distracting us from anxiety, anger, and sadness
- Food is a comforting tool; it comforts us when we are feeling sad or stressed
- Overeating sugary or unhealthy foods are associated with good times and celebrations
- Sugary and unhealthy foods are a reward
- Overeating can help one to overcome the fear that you won't manage to lose weight
- Food is a source of entertainment when one is feeling bored

- Ultimately, losing weight successfully with hypnosis requires that we assess these root causes, understand them, and finally reframe them. This is what hypnosis can do!

Chapter 5
Re-Program Your Mind

1)Visualization

If you want to reshape the reality of your life, start by visualizing how you want your ideal life to be. Our subconscious mind's primary language is emotions and images. Write a script of your perfect life and then play it like a movie in your imagination. The more detailed, vivid, and emotional you make it, the more your subconscious will think it is real because it cannot tell the difference. Remember the subconscious is your captive audience. You can transfer your ideas from your conscious imagination to your subconscious to make success happen for you. Do your visualization for 10 to 15 minutes daily.

• For visualization you can also use a vision board, which is covered in.

2) Affirmations

The trick to saying affirmations that work and can program your subconscious mind is confidence and perceived truth. Simply put, although our subconscious does not know the difference between real or fantasy, our affirmations should not raise internal objections because it is too farfetched. For example, if you are currently broke and unemployed, it might be a stretch for your subconscious to believe the affirmation "I'm going to be a billionaire by this December" as compared to "The ideal job is already mine. My finances are improving every day."

- Write affirmations that have corresponding feelings, focus on the positive, and have no opposing views.
- Face a mirror, take a deep breath and speak your affirmation a few times in the morning, noon, and evening. When saying your statement, focus on the meaning and feeling of your words.
- Another method is to write your affirmation several times on a piece of paper daily.
- Repetition and feelings are the key to reinforcing affirmations to your subconscious.

3) Listening to brainwaves audio program

Neuroscientists have discovered that different types of brain waves can influence our creativity, habits, behavior, thoughts, and moods.

There are 5 types of brain waves:

1. Beta brain waves are associated with our waking consciousness and are essential for our state of alertness, logic, and critical reasoning.
2. Alpha brain waves are present in deep relaxation, meditation, or dreaming states. This is also the optimal brain wave when we need to program our subconscious mind for success as it is when our imagination and visualization are at their peak.

3. Theta brain waves are present during light sleep, REM sleep, and meditation. These are also optimal waves for mind programming, vivid visualization, creativity, and insight.
4. Delta brain waves are the slowest brainwaves that happen during deep dreamless sleep and transcendental meditation. During these brain waves, our body is healing and regenerating.
5. Gamma brain waves are the fastest brainwaves which are associated with high-level processing and insight.

For subconscious programming, you can use either alpha or theta brain waves to help you while you are doing your visualization work. There are many apps and online audio programs that you can download such as Brain Waves - Binaural Beats, Brainwave Tuner Lite, Binality, edenBeats for Android and iPhone users.

4) Hypnosis

Typically, in hypnosis, a qualified hypnotist will put you in a relaxed and suggestible state before programming positive and empowering messages into your subconscious mind.

Techniques for Health

In we explained the emotions that harm our health and the mind-body connection where we feel a feeling and it activates specific neural pathways in our brain. Whether you're looking to improve a particular area of your health or your total wellbeing, the first step is to be aware of negative emotions that might be hampering your health. This step is like removing the weeds from your garden before you can start planting good seeds. The good news is once you have identified these negative emotions, you can work towards healthy subconscious programming.

- Be aware of your inner dialogue because every feeling, thought, and emotion carries energetic effects that can influence your body. For example, if you keep saying to yourself "I feel sad," it will cause stress, damage, and increase cortisol and adrenaline in your body. Imagine the long-term damage this does to your body if you do this repeatedly.

- Many diseases are manifested by our consistent toxic emotions and thoughts.

- Are you stuck in toxic emotions, such as anger or sadness, which are sending a negative feedback loop to your mind and body? Manage and take charge of your negative emotions otherwise they will control and deplete your mental strength.

- If you are currently undergoing treatment for any ailment, focus your mind on how the treatment or medication is going to help you get better. Let's say you are experiencing physical therapy for your bad knee. Instead of being passive and just going through the motions, you need to start seeing and believing that the treatment is indeed making your knee better. Use the power of your mind to expect your treatment to work.

- All sickness, be it the common flu or an incurable disease, can be reversed by releasing negative thoughts and replacing them with positive thoughts of health; healing through the mind works harmoniously with medicine.

- Our bodies respond to thoughts from our subconscious mind. Therefore, if you focus your thoughts on being healthy, you will create more health.

Steps:

- Ask for what you desire e.g., "I am healthy, and my body is perfect in every way"
- Every day, look at yourself in the mirror and say aloud your health affirmation "I am healthy, and my body is perfect in every way"
- Visualize your body in perfect health. Imagine yourself doing all the things you thought you couldn't do e.g.; your bad knee prevents you from running.
- To help you visualize better, cut out pictures of healthy-looking people that inspire you and paste it next to your mirror where you do your daily health affirmation
- Every day, try to do things that are relaxing and de-stressing to help you let go of toxic emotions and thoughts e.g., watching funny movies or playing with your children
- Be thankful and act like you already have a healthy body. If you want to accelerate your progress, keep a gratitude journal and write down three things you are grateful for before you sleep. The purpose is to let these positive thoughts sink into your subconscious and expand your awareness before you drift off to sleep.

- To keep your state of health, avoid people who are negative or focus too much on your illness
- Read (or listen) to books on health and wellbeing
- Lastly, believe and have faith that once you ask, your body is already whole.
- Suggested daily affirmations for health

E.g.

a) "I am getting stronger and healthier every day in every way."

b) "I am perfectly healthy and full of energy."

c) "I take good care of my body by eating healthy and nutritious food."

d) "I am filled with energy and physical stamina."

e) "I want wholeness and healing for my body."

f) "Healing power flows through my body in all ways."

g) "I am kind, loving and gentle to my body."

h) "I love food and food loves me back."

i) "I am at my perfect weight with a beautiful and healthy body."

Chapter 6
Self-Hypnosis Session

Simples Steps for Self-Hypnosis

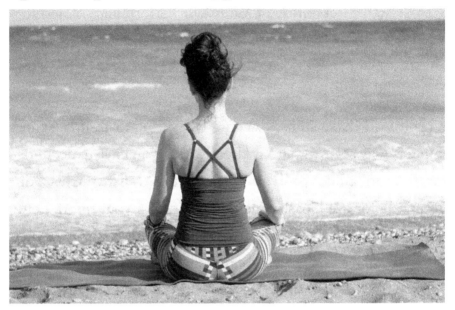

Now we will go over 10 succinct and straightforward steps to perform a successful and fruitful and positively productive session of self-hypnosis. I will list the steps first and follow up with a step-by-step breakdown featuring a brief and easy to understand the description of what each step should entail for you in your journey.

Step 1: Preparation of Self

Step 2: Preparation of Time

Step 3: Preparation of Space

Step 4: Preparation of Goal and Motive

Step 5: Relaxation of the Physical Body

Step 6: Relaxation of the Soul and the Mind

Step 7: Realization of Trance

Step 8: Active Repetition of Mantra or Performance of Script

Step 9: Preparation for Exiting the Trance State

Step 10: Returning to Earth

As you read those steps, I'm sure they bring forth images in your mind. It may seem apparent already what you have to do, and ideas for how to guide yourself through this self-hypnosis you are preparing for are blossoming like wildfire in your mind. Let us go more in-depth, to prepare further and become aware of all that you can do to make your self-hypnosis as comfortable and effective as your soul will wish, to better yourself in the most transformative way possible.

Step 1: Preparation of Self

So, as you are aware, one of the first and foremost goals is to become as relaxed as possible, before, during, and after entering the trance-state. Relaxation is the key that helps us enter the trance-state, and the trance-state further facilitates relaxation of the entire being both during the active self-hypnosis and afterward, for positive benefits of your being. To achieve the most successful self-hypnosis possible, we must first prepare ourselves, our minds and our physical bodies, for what we desire to achieve, a state of heightened relaxation in which we can become hyper-aware of the inner machinations of the mind, to achieve a closer union with them, to bond with them, and to converse with them on the most intimate level possible. The popularity of this music exists because people desire for sounds that will lull them into a more peaceful state. Maybe you would like to try something like this. Some people prefer silence; some people prefer quiet noise; a sort of hypnotizing drone that guides them into a more relaxed state of being. White noise, be it from a fan, a laundry machine, running water, or a white noise machine explicitly made for the purpose of filling the air with a light white noise, can also be useful for this purpose. Anything that has the desired effect on you will serve this purpose. Another thing, you can do is to drink a lovely herbal tea of your choosing; find a blend that is relaxing to you as an individual. Some common choices would be lavender-orange teas or chamomile teas. These will set a space internally for you to prepare yourself for entering your trance-state.

Step 2: Preparation of Time

It goes without saying that if an alarm clock goes on when you are in your trance-state, the effectiveness of your self-hypnosis session will be primarily inhibited. It is necessary, if you wish for an effective and transformative session of self-hypnosis, that you make sure a certain amount of time is allotted where you will be safe, secure, at peace, and uninterrupted by your daily responsibilities. Many things can get in the way of this. Common inhibitors of time include children, chores, spouses, day-to-day noise, and work. If you have children, maybe you can have a relative or a reliable babysitter, watch them for a certain amount of time. Perhaps you could ask your spouse to take the children out for an hour or two and explain to them your intentions of performing a transformative inner-journey that requires the utmost relaxation possible. Situations in which you have a significant burden of responsibility ironically are the types of situations that can make necessary long and fruitful journeys into self-hypnosis. It takes planning and care to make sure that, while all responsibilities are met, there is a designated and a specified time for you to go into your journey with the utmost confidence and care that you will be able to do what you need to do, and come out the other end as enlightened as possible.

Step 3: Preparation of Space

It also should go without saying that a crowded, busy subway station at peak times of the day is no place for you to go about your most effective journeys into self-hypnosis or the trance-like state. Place is of the essence. Just as your body temple must be totally clean and prepped and ready for the ascension, so must your surrounding area be prepared for you to feel as comfortable as possible to allow for the most successful transition into a strong and malleable trance-like state, allowing for the most successful self-hypnosis possible? As always, it is different for different people, depending on beliefs, religion, and personal comforts. Feel free to experiment and find what makes you most comfortable. No one knows how to make you as comfortable as possible, like yourself.

Trusting yourself is both one of the biggest keys and one of the biggest goals of self-hypnosis in general, so you must trust yourself here.

Step 4: Preparation of Goal and Motive

One of the critical factors of self-hypnosis is having a plan for what specific change or changes you wish to enact once having entered the trance state, and how you plan to achieve them. This is where the narratives you want to express, the prayers, or the mantra or mantras you wish to repeat to yourself, come into play. What do you hope to achieve in your self-hypnosis session? It is always different for different people and at different times. But there is still at least one goal, and preparation for achieving that goal is a must when it comes to performing a successful and fruitful and transformative self-hypnosis session. Imagine you are about to have an essential conversation with an essential person in your life. You are crossing a river one stepping stone at a time, putting one foot in front of the other, and you will make it across if you stay steady, attentive, and aware of your surroundings. Be calm, be collected, and be prepared for what you are about to do.

Step 5: Relaxation of the Physical Body

Now we begin. There are many schools of thought on the best ways to relax the body. One very common through-line in all of these is the act of deep, conscious breathing. Breath in, breath out, be aware of your breaths, be in control of each one of them. The goal here is mainly to become aware of every single voluntary and involuntary action of the physical body and slow it down. Feel your heartbeat. Be aware of it. Envision it slowing down. Relax. Expand the space and the length of each breath. Focus on some regions of the body and watch them become more and more still.

Step 6: Relaxation of the Soul and the Mind

So to relax the mind, we can perform a series of steps very similar to those shown when relaxing the body but carried over to another plane. Just as in relaxing the physical body our goal was to become totally aware of all voluntary and involuntary actions of the body, so as to slow them down to a point where they are more malleable and understandable, so too here, we must become aware of all the voluntary and involuntary actions of the mind, so as to slow them down to a point where they are more malleable and understandable. It is like slowly zooming in with a microscope, so things that were once small, almost imperceptible, become very large and monolithic. Our goal is to achieve a state of hyper-awareness.

Step 7: Realization of Trance

Now you are here, and you have willfully affected the realization of the trance-like state that is the initial aim of a good, useful session of proper self-hypnosis.

Don't be afraid to reach out and touch the light. Fully immerse yourself in this experience that you have prepared for. Know that you are achieving a fundamental and personal goal, and be glad and grateful and ecstatic and proud about where you are. Feel the ball of light at your core, your solar plexus, emanating out like a shining star, like the sun, like the soil. It may be orgasmic. You may be taken aback by the power you have tapped into, the infinite potential. Focus on the awareness of the self and see who you are.

Step 8: Active Repetition of Mantra or Performance of Script

Now you have journeyed into space. Speak.

Speak the words you wish to speak to yourself. Each repetition of the mantra will completely change the landscape that you have found yourself in seismic waves. You will feel a growing energy entirely under your control swarm over your entire being and beyond. You are in charge here. What you say goes. You are the ruler of this land, and you are going to take care of it well and make sure it is a prosperous paradise. Watch the negative thoughts, the images, the shadows, the memories you feared, the people you hate, the guilt, the pain, watch it shrivel into dust and evaporate before your very eyes, melted into oblivion by the sheer overwhelming power you have achieved.

Step 9: Preparation for Exiting the Trance State

Just as when you fully submersed, take a moment after you are done with your action to appreciate the beauty of what you are witnessing. Just be here now in this state. It is an eternal state. You will leave, and you will go back to the physical world, but this state will stay, untouched, timeless, waiting for you to return. This is heaven. Know that you are about to return, and you are about to feel very different than you have ever felt before. Embrace these differences. It may be odd and imperfect at first, but it is a learning experience. The physical reality still awaits you as always—a different eternal experience. The rest of your life will be spent juxtaposing these two very different and very real planes and finding the perfect balance where you are in absolute control, yet in total surrender and synchronicity.

Step 10: Returning to Earth

Open your eyes. Where are you? Who are you? You may feel like this is something equally new as the realm you have just left. But there is a feeling of familiarity. You are awakened to the infinite possibilities of life. You see that your perspective can change in endless ways, and with that change in perspective leads a portal to infinite different realties experienced through the multi-faceted crystal that is existence. You may be stunned. You will be changed.

Chapter 7
The Great Power of Meditation

Using Meditation to Stop, Calm, Rest and Heal Our Mind

About six months before I got my first job, I suffered a panic attack. I was not sure what it was, and I had no idea where it was coming from.

I was so worried about my new environment. The constant worry about meeting expectations kept me up at night. The idea of being among strangers and having to meet a required standard bugged me! How will I perform well? If I fail, how will I take care of my family?

To make things worse, panic drove me to try something that were not needed to fix my problem (problems that never really existed). I never once stopped to relax, to be calm, to rest, or even to heal myself. Instead, I was full of panic, worry, and constant fear. I was robbed of enjoying my job.

The above scenario depicts how many of us live our lives—in constant war and worry with ourselves. Our minds are in a steady state of chaos without us having any idea of how to calm them. This is why this part of this book is dedicated to teaching you how to take a step back, stop, pause, and heal your mind. This will allow you to revive your sense of peace and calmness.

The Buddha called this Samatha, the first part of the act of meditation. It is calming the mind and driving it to a state of peace (tranquility). Samatha involves:

• Putting a stop to harmful thought patterns.
• Bringing the mind to a peaceful state, even in difficult situations.
• Nourishing and resting the mind.
• Allowing the mind to heal and restore itself during deep pain or anguish.

Stopping

Just putting a stop to an unhelpful activity can be a mighty step. It is very beneficial yet so few know how to practice it.

For a week or two, try the following activity and note the difference in your life:

1. Have an alarm go off every 2-3 hours.
2. Once the alarm goes off, stop what you are doing and focus on our body.
3. Take note of the sensation that arises from your breathing.
4. Follow the length of your breath as it unfolds, pay attention to it as the air caresses your nostrils, circulating through your lungs, and returning out.
5. In case you get carried away, gently bring your thoughts back to our breathing.
6. Do this for 60 seconds, keeping your attention on your breath.

Stopping — the first part of Samatha — is not just about finishing in the physical sense. It also involves halting the influx of unhelpful thought patterns that drive us to rush through the day.

Generally, all humans possess powerful habit energy, which is the opposite of deliberate effort or free will. Looking at this in theory, it is like we should have the ability just to flip a switch and alter some parts of our lives. Unfortunately, it does not happen this way because our habit energy overpowers our willpower.

It is our habit of energy that pushes us around and fills us with unhelpful thoughts without our consent. This explains why many people do things that they do not want to do. This explains why a smoker will always resort to cigarettes despite knowing it is dangerous to their health.

This is where mindfulness comes in. It puts us back in the driver's seat of our lives and allows us to control what happens. Mindfulness brings with it an energy that directly involves us in our habit energy; we are aware of it and, just like that, we get to reduce its influence and control on our lives and activities.

With this mind, when next you give in to a bad habit, accept it mindfully and take note of the feelings and thoughts that come along with it. When you commit the act, what is the feeling that accompanies it?

These questions and process can help gain helpful insights that could help you calm your mind.

Calming

Calming involves letting go of strong emotions and calming the thoughts running through our minds.

There are many rewards for mindfulness- calming our thoughts is one of them. This is why mindfulness is so powerful in letting go of stress and anxiety. We do not need any special effort to calm our thoughts, although we have to build mindfulness into our habits.

Bear in mind, however, that the calming equation involves many things, with calming our thoughts as a part of it. We have to make an effort to handle strong emotions as they can be very harmful, especially in a restless mind. This is especially horrible when experiencing anxiety, as fear is one of the strongest emotions. If we don't handle these emotions, our progress will be minimal.

There is a method from Buddha (Buddha's approach for seeing deeply into our origin) to work through any negative emotion that baffles you consistently. The process is explained below:

1. Recognize - know that the emotions have surfaced with your mindfulness. "The fear has come." "I am afraid." These are the basics. You have got to acknowledge the emotions so that the remaining process will be useful.
2. Accept - rather than ignoring or trying to push the emotions away, accept them. Many of us resort to driving our destructive emotions away or assuming we are not there. This is a critical step as it alters our relationship with our feelings.

3. Embrace - with the spirit of compassion and self-love, come to terms with fear. Typically, our disposition towards these emotions is negative, which could be unhelpful. This step changes how we relate to our challenge, which sets us up for the natural healing process.

4. Look deeply - this step takes time. Now that we have accepted and come to terms with our fears, we need mindful meditation to get a deep insight into it. Where did the fear come from? What triggers it? What is the feeling that comes with it? While these questions are powerful and essential, don't fret too much. The primary step here is to be still, to meditate, and be mindful of the emotions as they arise. This is just like following a rabbit down its hole and keeping up with it to see how far it goes.

5. Realize - in other words, gain insights that come from looking deeply. This is what we want. Insight guides us to the part of ourselves where we are meant to be. We get ideas into what to do and avoid doing anything to change the situation.

6. This is a pretty long process, and I acknowledge that it can take some time. It is, however, useful in helping to get rid of strong emotions. This is a process that has worked for me in getting rid of emotional challenges and the negative energy radiating from them.

Resting

Rest is alien to most people. With the demands of everyday life, we hardly know how to relax our bodies and mind. A lot of people work late hours, even on weekends, which makes us prone to stress, anxiety, fatigue, and depression.

Resting involves caring for our body and mind through careful attention. This allows us to know when we are tired and when we need a time out, physically and mentally.

Lying down is not the only time we rest. The practice of meditation is pretty restful as well. Some activities that we can do to relax are:

- Sipping a glass of wine with mindfulness.
- Enjoying the sunset or sunrise while sitting and taking deep breaths.
- Taking a walk in the park while enjoying the elements of nature.
- Watering the flowers in our garden and being mindful of every moment.

Taking a break is not the primary time to take a rest. The critical thing to realize when it comes to rest, is that we should learn how to go about our daily activity with ease, joy, and calmness.

The Buddha advises walking a path in a simple, calm, and joyful way. The steps taken to stop and be calm will be of great help in accomplishing this. Also, practicing mindfulness of the body is a recommended tool. With the mindfulness of the body, we will always be in tune with our bodies. With time and practice, this will allow us to know when we are worn out when we need to take a step back and relax.

It is also critically important to pay proper attention to our time of sleep. To improve your quality of sleep, try the following tips:

- Avoid the screen and its reflection at least 2 hours before bed. Hence, TV sets, computers, tablets, mobile phones, etc. should be avoided.
- Get a warm glass of milk and drink it mindfully.
- Set and prepare your bedroom for sleep by reducing the temperature.
- Take a shower before getting into bed.

Healing

Living life in any random way without proper care is just setting ourselves up for negative experiences. By ignoring our bodies and not taking time to see a doctor, we might be opening ourselves up to a disease or ailment that could have been avoided.

In the same way, ignoring the happenings of our minds will only make it struggle more. This is, partly, a cause of depression—the worst state of anxiety and stress. When we finally take time to take care of ourselves, we would instead go for prescribed medications or a series of self-medication in a bid to keep ailments at bay. While I am not downgrading the effect of prescribed medication, it is of little or no use when it comes to taking care of the condition of the mind. Many people ignore the natural ability of the body and mind to heal.

Take an example of a wounded animal in a forest; the animal will look for a secluded place to rest and heal. They do not continue in their natural routine, running about and hunting. Humans can apply the same tactic, not just with the body but also with the mind. This makes much more sense if accompanied by additional treatment.

Imagine a disturbed body of water; we can't see to the bottom of the water. The same applies to a troubled mind; without seeing the cure, there is no way we will experience effective healing. With this, take time to learn and practice the process of stopping, being calm, and resting, which will bring clarity and natural healing.

Chapter 8
Guided Meditation

Meditation Exercise 1: Release of Bad Habits

Sit comfortably. Relax your muscles, close your eyes. Breathe in and breathe out. Do not cross your feet because this will lock you away from the desired experience. Hold your hands together to connect your logical brain hemisphere with your instinct.

Concentrate on your back now and notice how you feel in the bed or chair you are sitting in. Take a deep breath and let your stress leave your body. Now focus on your neck. Observe how your neck is joined to your shoulders. Lift your shoulders slowly. Breathe in slowly and release it. Feel how your shoulders loosen. Lift your shoulders again a little bit then let them relax. Observe how your neck muscles are tensing and how much pressure it has. Breathe in and breathe out slowly. Release the tension in your neck and notice how the stress is leaving your body. Repeat the whole exercise from the beginning. Observe your back. Notice all the stress and let it go with a profound breath. Focus on your shoulders and neck again. Lift up your shoulders and hold it for some moments, then rerelease your shoulders and let all the stress go away. Sense how the stress is going away. Now, focus your attention to your back. Feel how comfortable it is. Focus on your whole body. While breathing in, let relaxation come, and while you are breathing out, let frustration leave your body. Notice how much you are relaxed.

Concentrate on your inner self. Breathe slowly in and release it. Calm your mind. Observe your thoughts. Don't go with them because your aim is to observe them and not to be involved. It's time to let go of your overweight self that you are not feeling good about. It's like your body is wearing a bigger, heavier top at this point in your life. Imagine stepping out of it and laying it on an imaginary chair facing you. Now tell yourself to let go of these old, established eating and behavioral patterns. Imagine that all your past, fixed patterns and all the obstacles that prevent you from achieving your desired weight are exiting your body, soul, and spirit with each breath. Know that your soul is perfect as it is, and all you want is for everything that pulls away to leave. With every breath, let your old beliefs go, as you are creating more and more space for something new. After spending a few minutes with this, imagine that every time you breathe in, you are inhaling prank, the life energy of the universe, shining in gold. In this life force you will find everything you need and desire: a healthy, muscular body, a self that loves itself in all circumstances, a hand that puts enough nutritious food on the table, a loud voice to say no to sabotaging your diet, a head that can say no to those who are trying to distract you from your ideas and goals. With each breath, you absorb these positive images and emotions.

See in front of you exactly what your life would be like if you got everything you wanted. Release your old self and start becoming your new self. Gradually restore your breathing to regular breathing. Feel the solid ground beneath you, open your eyes, and return to your everyday state of consciousness.

Meditation Exercise 2: Forgiving Yourself

Sit comfortably. Do not cross your feet because this will lock you away from the desired experience. Hold your hands together to connect your logical brain hemisphere with your instinct. Relax your muscles, close your eyes.

Imagine a staircase in front of you! Descend it, counting down from ten to one.

You reached and found a door at the bottom of the stairs. Open the door. There is a meadow in front of us. Let's see if it has grass, if so, if it has flowers, what color, whether there is a bush or tree, and describe what you see in the distance.

Find the path covered with white stones and start walking on it.

Feel the power of the Earth flowing through your soles, the breeze stroking your skin, the warmth of the sun radiating toward you. Feel the harmony of the elements and your state of well-being.

From the left side, you hear the rattle of the stream. Walk down to the shore. This water of life comes from the throne of God. Take it with your palms and drink three sips and notice how it tastes. If you want, you can wash yourself in it. Keep walking. Feel the power of the Earth flowing through your soles, the breeze stroking your skin, the warmth of the sun radiating toward you. Feel the harmony of the elements and your state of wellbeing. In the distance, you see an ancient tree with many branches. This is the Tree of Life. Take a leaf from it, chew it, and note its taste. You continue walking along the white gravel path. Feel the power of the Earth flowing through your soles, the breeze stroking your skin, the warmth of the sun radiating toward you. Feel the harmony of the elements and your state of wellbeing. You have arrived at the Lake of Conscience, no one in this lake sinks. Rest on the water and think that all the emotions and thoughts you no longer need (anger, fear, horror, hopelessness, pain, sorrow, anxiety, annoyance, self-blame, superiority, self-pity, and guilt) pass through your skin and you purify them by the magical power of water. And you see that the water around you is full of gray and black globules that are slowly recovering the turquoise-green color of the water. You think once again of all the emotions and thoughts you no longer need (anger, fear, horror, hopelessness, pain, sorrow, anxiety, annoyance, self-blame, superiority, self-pity, guilt) and they pass through your skin and you purify them by the magical power of water. You see that the water around you is full of gray and black globules that are slowly obscuring the turquoise-green color of the water. And once again, think of all the emotions and thoughts you no longer need (anger, fear, horror, hopelessness, pain, sorrow, anxiety, annoyance, self-blame, superiority, self-pity, guilt) as they pass through your skin, you purify them by the magical power of water. And you once again see that the water around you is full of gray and black globules that are slowly obscuring the turquoise-green color of the water.

You feel the power of the water, the power of the Earth, the breeze of your skin, the radiance of the sun warming you, the harmony of the elements, the feeling of well-being.

You ask your magical horse to come for you. You love your horse, you pamper it, and let it caress you too. You bounce on its back and head to God's Grad. In the air, you fly together, become one being. You have arrived. Ask your horse to wait.

You grow wings, and you fly toward the Trinity. You bow your head and apologize for all the sins you have committed against your body. You apologize for all the crimes you have committed against your soul. You apologize for all the sins you committed against your spirit. You wait for the angels to give you the gifts that help you. If you can't see yourself receive one, it means you don't need one yet. If you did, open it and look inside. Give thanks that you could be here. Get back on your horse and fly back to the meadow. Find the white gravel path and head back down to the door to your stairs. Look at the grass in the meadow. Notice if there are any flowers. If so, describe the colors, any bush or tree, and whatever you see in the distance. Feel the power of the Earth flowing through your soles, the breeze stroking your skin, the warmth of the sun radiating toward you. Feel the harmony of the elements and your state of wellbeing. You arrive at the door, open it, and head up the stairs. Count from one to ten. You are back, move your fingers slowly, open your eyes.

Meditation Exercise 3: Weight Loss

Sit comfortably. Relax your muscles, close your eyes. Breathe in and breathe out. Do not cross your feet because this will lock you away from the desired experience. Hold your hands together to connect your logical brain hemisphere with your instinct.

Concentrate on your back now and notice how you feel in the bed or chair you are sitting in. Take a deep breath and let your stress leave your body. Now focus on your neck. Observe how your neck is joined to your shoulders. Lift your shoulders slowly. Breathe in slowly and release it. Feel how your shoulders loosen. Lift your shoulders again a little bit then let them relax. Observe how your neck muscles are tensing and how much pressure it has. Breathe in and breathe out slowly. Release the pressure in your neck and notice how the stress is leaving your body. Repeat the whole exercise from the beginning. Observe your back. Notice all the stress and let it go with a profound breath. Focus on your shoulders and neck again. Lift up your shoulders and hold it for some moments, then rerelease your shoulders and let all the stress go away. Sense how the stress is going away. Now, place your attention to your back. Feel how comfortable it is. Focus on your whole body. While breathing in, let relaxation come in, and while you are breathing out, let frustration leave your body. Notice how much you are relaxed.

Concentrate on your inner self. Breathe slowly and release it. Calm down your mind. Observe your thoughts. Don't go with them because your aim is to observe them and not to be involved. It's time to let go of your overweight self that you are not feeling good about. Imagine yourself as you are now. See yourself in every detail. Describe your hair, the color of your clothes, your eyes. See your face, your nose, your mouth. Set aside this image for a moment. See yourself in every detail. Describe your hair, the color of your clothes, your eyes. See your face, your nose, your mouth. Imagine that your new self-approaches your present self and pampers it. See that your new self-hugs your current self. Feel the love that is spread in the air. Now see that your present person leaves the scene and your new self takes its place. See and feel how happy and satisfied you are. You believe that you can become this beautiful new self. You breathe in this image and place it in your soul. This image will be always with you and flow through your whole body. You want to be this new self. You can be this new self.

Chapter 9
Affirmations and Subconscious Mind

The Power of Affirmations

Today is another day. Today is a day for you to start making a euphoric, satisfying life. Today is the day to begin to discharge every one of your impediments. Today is the day for you to get familiar with the privileged insights of life. You can transform yourself into improving things. You, as of now, include the devices inside you to do as such. These devices are your considerations and your convictions.

What Are Positive Affirmations?

For those of you who aren't acquainted with the advantages of positive affirmations, I'd prefer to clarify a little about them. A statement is genuinely anything you state or think. A great deal of what we typically report and believe is very harmful and doesn't make great encounters for us. We need to retrain our reasoning and to talk into positive examples if we need to change us completely.

An affirmation opens the entryway. It's a starting point on the way to change. When I talk about doing affirmations, I mean deliberately picking words that will either help take out something from your life or help make something new in your life.

Each idea you think and each word you express is an affirmation. The entirety of our self-talk, our interior exchange, is a flood of oaths. You're utilizing statements each second, whether you know it or not. You're insisting and making your background with each word and thought.

Your convictions are just routine reasoning examples that you learned as a youngster. The vast numbers of them work very well for you. Different beliefs might be restricting your capacity to make the very things you state you need. What you need and what you trust your merit might be unusual. You have to focus on your contemplations with the goal that you can start to dispose of the ones making encounters you don't need in your life.

Each time you blow up, you're asserting that you need more annoyance in your life. Each time you feel like a casualty, you're confirming that you need to keep on feeling like a casualty. If you believe that you think that life isn't giving you what you need in your reality, at that point, it's sure that you will never have the treats that experience provides for others-that is, until you change how you think and talk.

You're not a terrible individual for intuition, how you do. Individuals all through the world are quite recently starting to discover that our contemplations make our encounters. Your folks most likely didn't have the foggiest idea about this, so they couldn't in any way, shape, or form instruct it to you. They showed you what to look like at life in the manner that their folks told them. So no one isn't right. In any case, it's the ideal opportunity for us all to wake up and start to deliberately make our lives in a manner that satisfies and bolsters us. You can do it. I can do it. So how about we get to it.

I'll talk about affirmations as a rule, and afterwards, I'll get too specific everyday issues and tell you the best way to roll out positive improvements in your wellbeing, your funds, your affection life, etc. A few people say that "affirmations don't work" (which is an affirmation in itself) when what they mean is that they don't have a clue how to utilize them accurately. Some of the time, individuals will say their affirmations once per day and gripe the remainder of the time. It will require some investment for affirmations to work if they're done that way. The grumbling affirmations will consistently win, because there is a higher amount of them, and they're generally said with extraordinary inclination.

In any case, saying affirmations is just a piece of the procedure. What you wrap up of the day and night is significantly progressively significant. The key to having your statements work rapidly and reliably is to set up air for them to develop in. Affirmations resemble seeds planted in soil: poor soil, poor development. Fertile soil, bottomless event. The more you decide to think contemplations that cause you to feel great, the faster the affirmations work.

So, think upbeat musings, it's that straightforward. What's more, it is feasible. How you decide to believe, at present, is an only that-a decision. You may not understand it since you've thought along these lines for such a long time, yet it truly is a decision. Presently, today, this second, you can decide to change your reasoning. Your life won't pivot for the time being. Yet, in case you're reliable and settle on the decision regularly to think considerations that cause you to feel great, you'll unquestionably roll out positive improvements in each part of your life.

Positive Affirmations and How to Use Them

Positive affirmations are positive articulations that depict an ideal circumstance, propensity, or objective that you need to accomplish. Rehashing regularly these positive explanations, influences the psyche brain profoundly, and triggers it without hesitation, to bring what you are reworking into the real world.

The demonstration of rehashing the affirmations, intellectually or so anyone might hear, inspires the individual reworking them, builds the desire and inspiration, and pulls in open doors for development and achievement.

This demonstration likewise programs the psyche to act as per the rehashed words, setting off the inner mind-brain to take a shot at one's sake, to offer the positive expressions materialize.

Affirmations are extremely valuable for building new propensities, rolling out positive improvements throughout one's life, and for accomplishing objectives.

Affirmations help in weight misfortune, getting progressively engaged, concentrating better, changing propensities, and accomplishing dreams.

They can be helpful in sports, in business, improving one's wellbeing, weight training, and in numerous different zones.

These positive articulations influence in a proper manner, the body, the brain, and one's sentiments

Rehashing affirmations is very reasonable. Despite this, a lot of people do not know about this truth. Individuals, for the most part, restate negative statements, not positive ones. This is called negative self-talk.

On the off chance that you have been disclosing to yourself how miserable you can't contemplate, need more cash, or how troublesome life is, you have been rehashing negative affirmations.

Along these lines, you make more challenges and more issues, since you are concentrating on the problems, and in this way, expanding them, rather than concentrating on the arrangements.

A great many people rehash in their psyches pessimistic words and proclamations concerning the contrary circumstances and occasions in their lives, and therefore, make progressively bothersome circumstances.

Words work in two different ways, to assemble or obliterate. It is how we use them that decides if they will bring tremendous or destructive outcomes.

How to Use Meditation and Affirmations to Lose Weight

No Nonsense Weight loss affirmations the loss of weight is a great goal, but it sure helps you to get where you want to go if you have affirmations of weight loss. So why do weight claims help you get where you want to go?

Affirmations

Affirmations would help to wrap the mind around your goals and keep you focused as to where you want to be. So, when you're in its match, let's get those things moving.

Objective 1: Create the perfect healthy weight. The first bad part is to go there and achieve a certain ideal healthy weight. Don't talk about this. Even talk to your doctor about your perfect healthy level and do research. It is essential to raise an important subject at this stage. What is your ideal healthy weight, and assume you can't get there? It is safe to say that when it comes to appearance and obesity, society has set some rather strict standards.

When you see it, it is quite simple to define morbid obesity. This applies to a person who struggles with everyday life while carrying out basic tasks. But what happens to all of us if these tables that describe the criteria for the ideal height, weight, and body mass index of an individual cannot be matched? What are the rules if you are too thin?

Especially if you're not fit, there is a risk of being too thin. It would be far safer to be slightly overweight, but fit and healthy according to the scale. So, use common sense and never set your ideal weight by guess or because you think that this is the only weight you can take pleasure in. Focus your perfect weight on being healthy, but above all, a weight to keep you active and fit.

Objective 2: How I Am Going to Finish Objective 1.

You have your ideal healthy weight established, and you need to get there now. It's just another wasted opportunity if you don't. Next, ignore the lazy diet pills and crash diets that will take you back to where you started or worse. How is this a positive statement? See a fat farmer ever? I say one who works the farm every day. What makes the difference? The right to eat and physical activity. The body is designed for frequent and varied exercises. The main components of Objective 2 must be both aerobic and motivational tasks. For food, a balanced diet should be consumed, which takes approximately 1800-2800 calories a day for one person and less for a woman. Include as much organic food as possible to avoid fast food and processed food. Eat vegetables and fruits.

Objective #3-Believe it!

All right, we have Target 1 and Target 2 planned, now how can we convince ourselves that we're going to achieve these without falling off the car? You've been happy to ask about this. First, why do I have to believe it? Can I not just go?

Ever hear the phrase "been there"? That could only be the case, and how did it work? Not too good, perhaps, or you wouldn't be here now.

Chapter 10

Positive Affirmation for Weight Loss

Affirmations are statements made in order to really amplify a particular idea. Affirmations are certainly going to help take you through your diet. You are going to want to repeat these affirmations when you are feeling both positive and negative.

Whenever you feel like giving up or giving in, repeat these affirmations. Write them down, put notes around your home, and do whatever else is needed in order to keep you dedicated to your weight loss goals.

Affirmations for Losing Weight

This first set of affirmations is going to be great if you are interested in working out and dieting to lose weight. These affirmations can be said while you are working out or while you are eating.

When you are working out, affirmations are going to be helpful in order to get you to a place where you don't want to give up. If you feel like you just want to throw in the towel, try some affirmations to keep you focused on what matters most – not giving up.

Sometimes, we might mindlessly eat as well. This can be dangerous because it means that we are not focused on eating healthy. This could end up leading to overeating, or binge eating. If you want to control your portions, then these affirmations are helpful.

1. I know that I have control over whether or not I will lose weight.

2. I have the ability to get the body that I want.

3. It is possible to achieve my dreams.

4. I do not have to fantasize about my weight anymore. I have everything it takes to go through this process myself.

5. I have no guilt over my past choices.

6. Every decision I have made about my health has led me to where I am today.

7. I would not be who I am if it weren't for the struggle with my body that I have endured.

8. I am grateful for the battle that I have had with my body.

9. The challenges I've faced with my health have helped me to be more appreciative of what I have.

10. I might wish things were different with my body sometimes, but I know that I am grateful that they are the way they are now.

11. I am able to do so much with my body.

12. I know how to treat my body healthy so that I lose weight.

13. I am losing weight all the time, not just at certain moments.

14. As soon as I start to eat healthy, I feel lighter.

15. Whenever I work out, I feel lighter.

16. I am continually losing weight, and it is making my body healthier.

17. I know how to focus on healthy breathing.

18. My breathing helps me to lose weight even more.

19. When I am relaxed, I am happy.

20. When I am happy, I am losing weight.

21. I do not lose weight because I hate my body. I lose weight because I love my body.

22. I am exercising in order to take care of my health.

23. I am making healthy choices not just for me now, but for me later as well.

24. I am reaching the weight that I want each and every day.

25. I am continuously closer to getting the things that I have always wanted from my life.

26. I am healing myself when I lose weight.

27. My mind is improving just as much as my body is.

28. I am so lucky to have the amazing mind and body that I have.

29. I have essential parts in my body that I need to be grateful for.

30. My body could have less than what it has now, so I am grateful for the things that are present.

31. I am focused on pushing through my exercises.

32. Every time I want to give up exercising, I push forward because I know it will help me feel healthier.

33. Whenever I want to eat something that is bad for my body, I make sure to eat something healthy instead.

34. I do not torture my body with things that it cannot take.

35. I am putting my body through the challenges needed in order to get the results that I want.

36. I am focused on growing my body, not punishing it.

37. I want to teach my body healthy habits and that is precisely what I am doing.

38. I am helping my body be the best shape possible.

39. This is something that I deserve.

40. I am working hard and I deserve rewards.

41. I am not hard on myself when I don't meet a goal that I was hoping for.
42. I pick myself back up and keep moving on because I know that this is the most important thing that I can do.
43. I believe in myself and that is what matters the most.
44. I know how to get the healthy body that I want and there is nothing that is going to stop me.
45. I am capable of achieving my goals and I am the one that is in charge.

Affirmations for Feeling Better

When we are feeling gross, ugly, or discouraged, then we are not feeling great. If you want to really stick to a workout regime and lose weight, then it is crucial that you put an emphasis on feeling better. The better you feel, the easier it is going to be for you to have the confidence needed to make it to the gym, go for a walk, or attend the party.

Losing weight and getting healthy is essential in order for you to feel better, not just to look better. These affirmations are going to be useful in order for you to understand that as well.

Say these affirmations to yourself when you need to feel better, whether you are lethargic or self-conscious.

Listen to these frequently, even every day, in order to help remind you that you deserve to look good but feel even better.

1. I feel better and change myself based on the actions I choose to take.
2. I have everything I need in my life to feel good.
3. There is nothing that I can let make me feel bad at the moment.
4. I have what it takes to feel good all the time.
5. I am entirely in control of my emotions.
6. Others might do things that make me feel bad but I am in control of how much I let these things affect me.
7. I deserve to feel good all the time.
8. Others know that I deserve to feel good.
9. Other people like being around me.
10. Other people want me to feel good.
11. I want others to feel good. We should all be feeling good.
12. It is my positive attitude that helps me to feel even better.
13. I am always excited and ready to start a new day.
14. I look forward to what adventures might be waiting for me tomorrow.
15. There is nothing in my life that scares me or holds me back from doing what I want.
16. I have the confidence needed to accomplish my wildest dreams.
17. I believe in myself and that is what is going to power me through and help me find the things that I have been looking for.
18. I have no problem deciding what I should do because I always know what is best.
19. I know how to listen to my body, and I can tell whether it is feeling good or bad.
20. I have so much joy that it overflows to others.

21. I am able to spread how good I feel because I have so much positive energy.

22. Even when I am in pain, it does not affect my mood.

23. I appreciate the pain because I know it is presenting me with a healthy struggle.

24. Everything that I will ever need is something that I already have.

25. I don't have to be worried about anything making me feel bad because I have the power to change my perspective.

26. I feel good and, therefore, I look good.

27. I look good and, therefore, I feel good.

28. There is nothing else I need moving forward to make me happy. Everything that does make me happy is going just to be an added benefit.

29. I know what it takes to feel good.

30. I make right decisions all the time so that I feel good all the time.

31. I only include positive habits in my life that will help me to feel better overall.

32. There is no one that feels as good as I do.

33. I care about how I feel because that is what matters first.

34. I believe in myself and that helps me to feel better.

35. Whenever I am feeling down, I know how to turn my mood around and feel better.

36. Everything that has happened bad in my life has taught me how to feel better.

37. I am not afraid of what might be out there because I know that no matter how bad it might be, I will still be able to feel good.

38. There are things I can't control in my life, but I know how to do what is essential so that I am in control.

39. I defeat challenges easily because I feel good about myself.

40. I am able to stand up for what I think is right and fight for a good purpose.

41. I always feel good because I choose to, even when things are tough.

42. I know that feeling bad does me no good, so I will always focus on how I can feel good.

Chapter 11
Repetition Like a Mantra

What are Mantras and How, For What Can We Use Them?

There are a lot of anxiety-inducing situations every day such as an essential job interview, asking the boss for a pay raise, giving a lecture in front of a bunch of people, and so on. Calm breathing often turns out to be insufficient, especially in a stressful emergency situation. In this case, we need to apply another approach, the method of mantra.

What are mantras - how and for what can we use them?

There are a lot of anxiety-inducing situations every day - an important job interview, asking the boss for a pay raise, giving a lecture in front of a bunch of people, and so on. Calm breathing often turns out to be insufficient, especially in a stressful emergency situation. In this case, we need to apply another approach: the method of mantra.

10 Essentials You Need to Know About Mantras

1. The hidden possibilities of mantras

The strength of mantras honed by ancient Indian sages over many decades is concentrated, even in their ability to influence the physical level. "Mantras are like different doors that lead to the same end: each mantra is unique and thus leads to the same wisdom: to recognize that everything is one. That is, every mantra has the potential to unleash the veil of illusion and dispel the darkness. " (Deva Premal)

2. The language of mantras and their meanings

The style of mantras is Sanskrit, which is no longer considered a living language on the planet, but it is called the 'mother tongue'. We all relate to this in the same way as our language is a cellular language, a code that we understand at a profound level. It vibrates in us something that no other language or sound can. It is a universal, cellular voice that unites us, no matter our belief system, our nationality, and our religion. You can find translated mantras, but the sounds themselves are sufficient to bring about the beneficial effects. Mantras contain deep, concentrated wisdom, meaning much more than the sum of individual words. It is therefore almost impossible to translate them accurately without losing some deeper meaning. Therefore, let us consider the translation as a guide and make the mantras work on their own.

3. The power of intention

As something is necessarily lost in the true meaning of translation, the power of our intention is significant. It is good to have a firm purpose and a strong focus inside, but in fact, the effect that the mantra exerts on us is the most important. This is the true meaning of the mantra to every person who uses it. For each mantra, you will find a phrase called "Inner Focus", which broadly covers the intent of that mantra, but of course, you can also formulate an individual intent.

4. Keep the mantra with you all day

There are countless ways to make mantras part of our lives. I often carry a mantra with me all day. I would like to encourage you to do so! Carry the mantra with you throughout the day, and whenever you think of it, come back to it, the mantra being the last thing you think of before going to sleep. This is how you can truly commit to a mantra and the specific focus or theme that the mantra represents.

5. It's not necessary to chant the mantras aloud.

Mantras do not necessarily have to be heard out loud. Understanding this can be a real breakthrough because it means you could carry the mantra on your own without actually chanting. So if there is a situation where you feel you need to sing the mantra out loud, concentrate on pushing it inward, carry it with you, and hold it in your being, your mind, your heart - this is the root of mantra practice when we connect with the Spirit.

6. Chant your mantras 108 times

108 is considered a very favorable number in the Vedas. According to the scriptures, we have 72,000 lines of energy in our body (the nadis), of which there are 108 main channels of energy or major nadi that meet in the sacred heart. When a mantra is chanted 108 times, all energy channels are filled with vibrations of sound.

7. In what position should we mantra?

I recommend a comfortable position for most mantras, one with a straight back; we can relax and yet remain alert. A position that allows us presence. Because of this, a lying position is not ideal, it is harder to sing and we risk falling asleep while doing it.

8. Contemplation

Before each mantra, let's reflect on the topic of that mantra: what does it mean in our lives, do we need it, can we develop in that area, etc.? What can we sacrifice to make this quality more fully manifest in our lives? Thinking through these steps helps to refine our focus further and deepen our practice.

9. The most important "element" of the mantra is silence.

Be aware that the most important "element" of the mantra that we reach through the mantra is the silence. This is seemingly a paradoxical thing: the silence after singing is what our soul dives into and is reborn. This silence represents the transcendent, the eternal, the reality, and understanding or achieving this is the ultimate goal of mantra practice.

10. Importance of repetition and practice

The essence of mantra practice is not to get over it quickly and then return to our usual daily routine. The point is to practice and to integrate the mantras into our lives. Wherever we go, whatever we do, the mantras accompany us. This is the benefit of right mantra practice. It helps and supports the path of our lives. The power of mantras is multiplied by repetition and devotional practice. The more pleasure we can bring into our practice, the more pleasure we get. Like real friends, mantras can help you through times of need and stress.

How do we use mantras in everyday life?

The method is simple! We need to talk to ourselves - of course, what we say matters. I may surprise you by saying that it's enough to repeat only three words in every situation when you feel under pressure. These three words are: "I am excited."

Yes, I know, it is not what you have expected from me. You may wonder why you should use a statement that is not so 'positive'. Harvard University published a study in the Journal of Experimental Psychology, in which scientists claim that striving to overcome anxiety may not be the best solution in such situations. Instead of trying to calm ourselves down, it can be more useful to transform stress into a powerful and positive emotion, such as excitement. Because positive feelings produce quite similar physical symptoms as anxiety, hence, we wouldn't have great difficulties switching the stress to excitement. Enthusiasm is a positive emotion; besides, it is easier to cope with. The study also recalls earlier research that mild anxiety can even be a motivator for specific tasks. So, it is worth using the energy generated by stress to increase our efficiency, instead of trying our best to suppress it. To turn fear-based anxiety into a positive feeling, repeat for 60 seconds to yourself, "I am excited." This mantra "redraws" the picture of a stressful situation into something we happen to be waiting for - which is far less exhausting than trying to calm ourselves down.

Using different mantras is very important to me, and I use them daily for my meditations or just for relaxation. You can also use them whenever you are sad, or you don't know where you belong to what you have to do with your life. They help you to see through and view yourself. If you have been to a place where people have been singing or chanting, you will know how much power and energy there is in a particular word.

One of the best-known mantras is "Aum" or "Oum." It is found among Hindus but also in Buddhism. Followers believe this mantra purifies the soul and helps to release negative emotions. This mantra is also known as a sign of the "quick eye" chakra.

If you want to reach the best result, sing AUM loudly so that its sound vibrates in your ears and soaks your entire body. It will convince your outer sense, give you greater joy and a sense of success. When singing AUM loudly, "M" should sound at least three times as long as "AU". When repeating "AUM", imagine that life energy, divine energy flows through you through the crown chakra. The breath that flows through your nose is very limited. But if you can imagine that there is a large opening at the top of your head, and life energy, cosmic energy is flowing into your body through that opening, you will undoubtedly be able to accelerate the purification of your nature, strengthen your aspiration and hunger for God, Truth, Light, and Salvation.

Chapter 12

Sharp Your Mind to Shape Your Body

Perfect Mind, Perfect Weight

Perfect thoughts and ideal weight." The term may seem like a fantasy to you. Which is the ideal mind or ideal weight? They're the realistic conditions you'll be able to utilize as you pursue fat reduction. "Realistic?" You inquire. "How can anything be 'ideal,' let alone my burden and my ideas about my burden?" Well, recall what we said about the strength of believing and belief. Is it serving your curiosity to desire or hope to anything less than perfection on your own? Indulge us for some time as we clarify why you're able to think your mind and burden because "perfect."

Perfect fat is your weight that's ideal for you. It's the weight that's attainable and consistent with everything you need and precisely what you're ready to give yourself and accept yourself. More to the point, your ideal weight provides you with the healthy entire body, the human body which goes effortlessly, and also the one where you are feeling great about yourself and joyful. And what're ideal thoughts? You presently have a mind. It's flawless. But there can be a few ideas in that ideal thought of yours who are providing you with undesirable outcomes. There can be something that you keep in your mind, possibly habits or routines, which provide you with undesirable outcomes. However, you may use your ideal head to match your ideas to offer you precisely what you desire. It's possible to use your head to accomplish the bodyweight that you desire.

In the Twinkling of an Eye

Your current body is the consequence of your ideas and beliefs. You've behaved out these ideas and beliefs by your lifestyle, which generated your current weight. You haven't made any errors, regardless of what you may be thinking of yourself; instead, you've just experienced undesirable outcomes. These undesirable effects are an immediate effect of misaligned ideas and beliefs about yourself, which are very patterns of behavior or lifestyle. The Rapid Weight Loss Diet is all about utilizing your perfect thoughts

To align your ideas to provide you with the results you desire. You honestly can use your head to accomplish the bodyweight you desire. Let's take a look at a few of the learning which has occurred in your life which has let you know where you're now together with your body weight. Do you wake up one afternoon, and you had been using the additional pounds? Or could it be a slow accumulation with time? Or perhaps you've understood nothing else as early youth. Whatever the situation, there are lots of factors that made your body:

- Food options

- Eating customs

- That the self-critic in you

- Economic history

- Psychological history

- Impact of household

- Impact of buddies

- Cultural heritage

These and several other variables were discovered in your life and eventually became the beliefs, which subsequently became routines of activity that generated your body. In other words, consider what you did understand about your youth about eating and food.

- What kinds of grocery stores did your household buy?
- What foods did your kids cook, and were they typically ready?
- Can you eat only at home or often grab food?
- Have you been served fresh, healthy, high-calorie foods, or can you eat mainly processed and extremely processed foods, fried foods, and "junk" foods?
- Was there aware focus on nutrition, or has been there any irresponsible disregard for that which your household ate?
- What did you find out about eating mindfully?
- Were you educated that healthful food options led to healthy bodies?
- Did anybody teach you how you can understand what's healthy food and what's not?
- Are your meals selections based on which tasted or seemed high or priceless?
- Can your loved ones or college instruct you about healthy lifestyles and audio nourishment, or has been the "nutrition education" through TV advertisements and food makers' advertising?

What exactly did you learn as a kid? What're your beliefs about eating food, along with your entire body? Analyze your own socioeconomic or socio-cultural roots and see if they had an effect on the way and what you've learned to consume. Over thirty-five Years Back, sociological research pointed out weight issues in the working and lower class according to their intake patterns of what's been known as "poverty-level foods," like hot dogs, canned meats, and processed luncheon meats.

Cultural groups also have been analyzed to understand their nutritional patterns and meals, like eating with lard or ingesting a diet of fried and high-fat foods, can lead to higher body fat loss. These influences can readily be accepted because they're "regular" into the category of course. Then let's take a look in the teen years. During adolescence, are there some changes in your weight loss? Just as a boy, have you been invited to pile more food in your plate? "Look at him, consume! Certainly, he will develop to a large guy!" (There's a telling metaphor) Or are you currently admonished to eat? When you're a budding young woman, did a Smart girl take you under her wing and then discuss with you that the marvel of menses and the wonderment of body modifications, such as the organic growth in body fat with all the evolution of breasts and broader hips?

Were you conscious during puberty which unless the body improved body fat by 22 per cent, it wouldn't correctly grow and create menses? Or was that "hushed up" within an awkward improvement? It was likely during adolescence which you heard there's a stigma involving obese individuals. Ponder the encounters and influences which are forming your body. In high school, the athletes at college sports have always been a healthful weight and are the cheerleaders and homecoming queens.

What ancient beliefs regarding your popularity and self-image could have formed from your social interactions in high school? What did you understand about physical activity, and what customs did you produce? Have you been introduced to physical activity as part of a healthful lifestyle, through family or sports outings of walks or hikes? Or was that the blaring TV a regular fixture, enticing everybody to the sofa? Next is a matter which most people have never been aware of throughout their development.

As you're growing up, has been that the attention of self-care based on trendy clothes, makeup, and hairstyles, or about healthful food, routine physical activity, along with spiritual and intellectual nourishment? What about today? Spend a couple more minutes writing down the aspects that appear to be accurate for you in the past couple of decades. What influences and experiences formed the ideas, which turned in the beliefs that turned into your body?

After high school, you moved away from the house. Suddenly you're no more captive to your family lifestyle. Can you be aware of your options, or can you start eating with blow off? If you input into a close connection, just what compromises or arrangements about foods and physical activity did you input into too? Most associations develop from similar pursuits, including food preferences and eating styles. In the end, the relationship comprises eating routines and tastes, which are a consequence of compromise.

Have your connections encouraged smart food choices and healthy eating? Maybe you've experienced pregnancy. Can you learn the way to get a wholesome pregnancy and then nourish a healthy infant within you? Or did you put in pounds? After giving birth, how did your lifestyle assist you in recovering your typical fat or suppressing it? If you were more active in the league or sports games, did your livelihood or family duties take priority and eliminate these physical fitness tasks from your regular? Can you correct exercise and diet so, or even did the fat begin to collect? Did an accident, injury, or disease happen that disrupted a standard physical action that has been supportive of healthy fat?

Because you can see, the way you got to where you're now was no crash. You heard from the folks about you--or you also consumed out of the surroundings --the best way to create food decisions, the way to eat, and the way to look after yourself emotionally and physically. Whether the thoughts you heard were tremendous and healthy or not so high and not as healthy, they became your own beliefs, and eventually became you and the own human body because it is now. Bear in mind, and you didn't do something wrong; however, you need to experience the outcomes of eating and living, which have been consistent with your ideas and beliefs.

Through time, what's been your answer to individuals and their opinions about your weight loss, bad or good? Can you go out and purchase a fantastic pair of sneakers, or do you consume to facilitate psychological distress? Maybe you even heard the latter response on your youth.

Did your mom ever provide you with a plateful of food to comfort you when you're miserable? These are learned answers, and they may be unlearned and replaced with new answers and routines to make your ideal weight. Just ask, "Just how long does this happen?" We inform you, "In the twinkling of the eye" For the minute that you understand that you need it sufficient to get anything to possess it, it's completed. You've just altered the management of highly efficient energy in you which will be directed at figuring out how to attain the outcome which you need: your ideal weight.

Your Perfect Mind Relearning

It's simple to comprehend how you got or "heard" to contemplate over your ideal weight. And it'll be simple to create new decisions, to relearn new routines, and also to make new and much more healthful habits. How can we learn? We understand by mimicking another individual, analyzing books with different tools and practicing the activities that create the outcomes we all seek. The best and lasting learning entails repetition and practice. The best way to practice is essential. Pretend for a minute that you're a violinist. You're searching for a grand symphony operation in New York.

The critical thing is that you're giving your focus on practicing correctly.

Chapter 13
Heal Your Relationship with Food

As you can see, the desire to reduce sugar is not easy. It becomes not only our habit, but we also become physically dependent on it. It disturbs our health and even our overall functioning as individuals in the society.

A Simple and Magical Solution Does Not Exist.

Yes, there are foods that are healthy and which can replace sugar, but it takes discipline and a change of lifestyle.

In the morning, after a night when you don't eat, your blood sugar level is the lowest and we should eat a meal that provides a constant increase of sugar to avoid hunger attacks. It is best that this meal contains a combination of protein and complex carbohydrates (bread, pasta) because they are digested slowly.

This is about enough for me to start the day. Fruit also causes relatively rapid rises in blood sugar, and therefore it might be better to eat it in the afternoon after lunch, but with a gap as it is quickly digested and absorbed best on an empty stomach. This will help in the afternoon when our energy is lowered, and will not have such a yo-yo effect on blood sugar as chocolate or ice cream.

Chapter 14
We Shall Talk Here About Breakfast in Order to Really Know Why It Is So Important.

Most people forget that breakfast is the most important meal of the day, I was among them until recently too. Believe me when I say that I never forgot about lunch, even only to eat something quickly. Basically, it is more of an abundant meal to make up for the lack of breakfast, and usually was full of fat and sugar that could help me. As I already said, this meal leads to a rapid decline of satiety and blood sugar, and I would often eat an abundant snack. The fact that I went to the gym was in vain for me.

Although this daily regime diet is wrong, long ago we gained the habits and if you want to reduce the desire for sugar, this is the first thing you have to change.

We neglect breakfast because we are in a hurry to rush to work, to school, to catch a bus, or because we just want to sleep a little longer almost every morning, or finally because we do not want to prepare a meal every morning. No matter what the reason for this behavior, the fact remains that all the food experts recommend changing our consumption habits. We are working hungry, and we rest when we are full. This is our greatest problem.

Breakfast, which most of us don't practice too much, should be fat and caloric. The day should start strong, and we should be fed to handle the physical and mental efforts that await us.

Let us not forget that our breakfast should provide about a quarter of daily needs in energy, building, and protective substances, which are the main components of our food. Most people do just the opposite: Working hungry, resting when full, which is quite wrong. Breakfast should be rich and full of calories, to start the day strong, fed, and that way to satisfy the physical and mental efforts set by our workplace. All other meals, no matter what you are eating are upgrades and additions.

I personally do not avoid meat. I actually extremely enjoy it, but I try to have still a lunch or dinner which will not be a caloric bomb, even when I eat meat this is why I usually combine it with vegetables and spices. In this way, my meals do not only get healthier, but a lot tastier too.

Try avoiding processed meat, such as for example salami, which is full of preservatives. I always try to find fresh meat and fresh vegetables and not to have a monotonous diet.

In essence, treat your body as you treat your mobile phone. In the morning before you leave home, you charge it, to have plenty of power, and then if necessary, you recharge it.

When you combine this developed habit of eating with physical activity and a bit of sports, believe me, you will not reach for sweets or sugar. If you regularly provide your body with everything it needs, you will have no more cravings for sugar or for anything else.

The Secret Is In Moderation

What I discovered during my journey and my research is that the secret to healthy living without sugar is actually moderation and balance. It is necessary to examine yourself and to know your needs and how to meet them effectively.

You do not need to exaggerate anything. If you feed your body well, it will send you signals exactly when and what you need. Just listen to your body, and everything will be ok.

Why do I point this out? I emphasize this because I have observed that often we exaggerate healthy things, which eventually leads to the same effect as before.

When you tell someone that a particular food or ingredient is healthy for him, he can often overdo it and eat or drink only that, or some insane amounts of it. This can best be seen in the case of fresh fruit juice.

We all know that fresh fruit juice is healthy, and that we should drink it. But people often exaggerate this. Many people think that fresh juices are good in all quantities and are harmless. However, this is not the case. Same juice can help one person, and also harm the other.

Fresh juices are a bad choice for some diseases. So if you have a peptic ulcer, gastritis and pancreatitis you should not drink the juice of lemons, oranges, apples, currants, or cranberries. They contain many organic compounds, which increase the acidity of the stomach, which can cause discomfort and pain. Consumption of grape juice should be limited if you have diabetes. It contains too much glucose and calories. Remember, many fresh juices also have laxative properties.

After all, they are not healthy for your sugar cravings or for your body if you consume too much. Let's say that you get a full glass of orange juice, for which you have to squeeze around four average oranges. If you eat four oranges, you would likely be full and it will be a little hard for your stomach. Both of those have the same energy value, but you just did not notice this, because you just drank it in two gulps.

You should treat the same way all the sweets that may contain unhealthy sugars. Nobody is saying that you should not eat them at all, but you should know when you have consumed enough, and you need to know to then how to act accordingly.

As I've already said so far, the struggle is for your own health, and therefore happiness begins with a good scare. Fear is one of the biggest motivators.

Good Company Instead Of Good Food

It's trite to say that humans are social animals. We all know this.

What's odd is that, notwithstanding our knowledge that we are social creatures, we often live remarkably isolated lives.

Humans evolved in small groups of people all of whom were related to and knew each other intimately. The worst fate that could befall an early human at the hands of his fellows was ostracism from the tribe. It meant almost certain death.

From an evolutionary standpoint, we have come to associate being alone with danger. It is a state which is inherently stressful for us, particularly when it is protracted.

Solitary confinement, which is used to punish prison inmates, is punitive for this reason.

But there are positive benefits to associating with other humans which also have their roots in our evolutionary history.

In a tribe, with individuals to whom you are related, and have known all your life, there's an acceptance which goes beyond mere kinship.

No matter how embarrassing, foolish or misguided a tribal member's behavior may be on a given day, she at least has the benefit of having seen every other member of the tribe on their worst day as well.

What's more, the other members are readily available for comfort and support.

An anthropologist studying a tribal people in Papua New Guinea once observed a woman, after an argument with her husband, begin to dismantle their dwelling out of anger.

Halfway through the task she realized the folly of this and to save face took the leaves which had formed the roof of the hut down to the stream and washed them as though that had been her purpose all along.

Without saying a word, either to her or one another, the other women in the tribe proceeded to take leaves off the roofs of their own huts and bring them to the stream to wash.

Our modern lives stand in stark contrast to the lives enjoyed by our tribal ancestors. We did not evolve to live in the comparative isolation which we have come to take for granted.

So it's not surprising that loneliness is a common trigger for emotional eating.

If you feel drawn to any of the social food alternatives suggested below it's a safe bet that loneliness, isolation, or a feeling of disconnect from others is at the root of your emotional distress.

Social food alternative.

1. Call a friend/visit a friend. We tend to spend a lot of time on social media these days which creates the illusion that we are connected to people. In fact, spending time alone — whether spending it reading about the lives of other people or doing something else — is still spending time by ourselves. It doesn't give us the connection we crave.

Social media also tends to cause us to compare ourselves to others, rather than connect with them. People post, on Facebook or elsewhere, the highlights of their lives rather than their lows. If all we do is look at social media, we get the impression that everyone else is having a better time than us.

Calling a friend, or visiting a friend or friends, permits us to be able to connect with them and share our problems, reciprocating by allowing them to share theirs. Even just being in the presence of a friend can be calming.

As social creatures, we are soothed when we are around others whom we know and trust. Spending time talking to a friend, or in the presence of a friend or group of friends, soothes our primitive brain and reduces the anxiety it produces.

Friends mirror us, validate us, and support us just by being there for us. There's an old saying, "if you wish to have a friend, be one." Calling or visiting a friend gives us the opportunity to show us that we are there for them, while we also reap the rewards of friendship.

Chapter 15
Mindful Eating Habits

Mindfulness is a simple concept that states that you must be aware of and present in the moment. Often, our thoughts tend to wander, and we might lose track of the present moment. Maybe you are preoccupied with something that happened or are wondering about something that might happen. When you do this, you tend to lose track of the present. Mindful eating is a practice of being conscious of what and when you eat. It is about enjoying the meal you eat while showing some restraint. Mindful eating is a technique that can help you overcome emotional eating. Not just that, it will teach you to enjoy your food and start making healthy choices. As with any other skill, mindful eating also takes a while to inculcate, but once you do, you will notice a positive change in your attitude toward food. In this, you will learn about a couple of simple tips you can use to practice mindful eating in your daily life.

Reflection

Before you start eating, take a minute and reflect upon how and what you are feeling. Are you experiencing hunger? Are you feeling stressed? Are you bored or sad? What are your wants and what do you need? Try to differentiate between these two concepts. Once you are done reflecting for a moment, you can now choose what you want to eat, if you do want to eat and how you want to eat.

Sit Down

It might save some time if you eat while you are working or while traveling to work. Regardless of what it is, you must ensure that you sit down and eat your meal. Please don't eat on the go, instead set a couple of minutes aside for your mealtime. You will not be able to appreciate the food you are eating if you are trying to multitask. It can also be quite difficult to keep track of all the food you eat when you are eating on the go.

No Gadgets

If all your attention is focused on the TV, your laptop or anything else that comes with a screen, it is unlikely that you will be able to concentrate on the meal that you are eating. In fact, when your mind is distracted, you tend to indulge in mindless eating. So, limit your distractions or eliminate them if you want to practice mindful eating.

Portion your Food

Don't eat straight out of a container, a bag or a box. When you do this, it becomes rather difficult to keep track of the portions you eat, and you might overindulge without even being aware of it. Not just that, you will never learn to appreciate the food you are eating if you keep doing this.

Small Plates

We are all visual beings. So, if you see less, your urge to eat will also decrease. It is a good idea to start using small plates when you are eating. You can always go back for a second helping, but this is a simple way to regulate the quantity of food you keep wolfing down.

Be Grateful

Before you dig into your food, take a moment and be grateful for all the labor and effort that went into providing the meal you are about to eat. Acknowledge the fact that you are lucky to have the meal you do, and this will help create a positive relationship with food.

Chewing

It is advised that you must chew each bite of food at least thirty times before you swallow it. It might sound tedious, but make it a point to chew your food at least ten times before you swallow. Take this time to appreciate the flavors, textures and the taste of the food you are eating. Apart from this, when you thoroughly chew the food before swallowing, it helps with better digestion and absorption of food.

Clean Plate

You don't have to eat everything that you serve in your plate. I am not suggesting that you must waste food. If you have overfilled your plate, don't overstuff yourself. You must eat only what your body needs and not more than that. So, start with small portions and ask for more helpings. Overstuffing yourself will not do you any good, and it is equivalent to mindless eating.

Prevent Overeating

It is important to have well-balanced meals daily. You shouldn't skip any meals, but it doesn't mean that you should overeat. Eat only when you feel hungry and don't eat otherwise. Here are a couple of simple things you can do to avoid overeating. Learn to eat slowly. It isn't a new concept, but not many of us follow it. We are always in a rush these days. Take a moment and slow down. Take a sip of water after every couple of bites and chew your food thoroughly before you gulp it down. Don't just mindlessly eat and learn to enjoy the food you eat. Concentrate on the different textures, tastes, and flavors of the food you eat. Learn to savor every bite you eat and make it an enjoyable experience. Make your first-bit count and let it satisfy your taste buds. Now is the time to let your inner gourmet chef out! Use a smaller plate while you eat, and you can easily control your portions. Stay away from foods that are rich in calories and wouldn't satiate your hunger. Fill yourself up with foods that can satisfy your hunger and make you feel full for longer. If you have a big bowl of salad, you will feel fuller than you would if you have a small bag of chips. The calorie intake might be the same for both these things, but the hunger you will feel afterward differs. The idea is to fill yourself up with healthy foods before you think about junk food. While you eat, make sure that you turn off all electronic gadgets. You tend to lose track of the food you eat while you watch TV.

Chapter 16
How to Practice Every Day

The first thing you need to do when it comes to managing time is to look at yourself. Look at what you're trying to get done. Look at the goals that you have and aspirations that you have. Look at how you can use your time in order to make things better. If you look at yourself and see that you need a certain amount of time in order to make sure that you get things done, you'll see that you need to have that time in order to achieve your goals. Looking at the broad picture can help.

The next thing, once you've looked at the broad picture, is to make a plan. A plan for this is the overall goal that you have and how in the world you're going to get to it. Some goals are huge, such as trying to run the marathon or getting to a goal weight, but you can achieve them. You should look at everything that you need to do in order to achieve the goal that you have. It's not something that will take five minutes to do, but if you have a plan it'll make things easier. You want to have an exact set of steps that you'll need to do in order to get to the state that you want to be in. If you want to run the marathon, plan out how you're going to run it. Go through the exact steps, and you'll soon see the overall things that you need to do in order to get to that point. It might look daunting at the moment, but if you work at this, you'll see that the dreams that you have can become a reality if you follow the overall game plan that can help with your goals.

The next thing is to make a monthly plan. You look at exactly what you want to accomplish this month. It can be goals that are big or small, but don't bite off more than you can chew. Thing about what you can realistically do in order to hit a certain goal. You have to look at what you need to change in order to accomplish all of those things. A monthly plan allows you to change the way things go, and you can also change the way life goes as time passes. A monthly plan will keep you on track and motivated to keep on going with the goals that you have in mind.

Next, think of how the goal can be divided into four weeks. Dividing it down and making sure that you have a good plan in order to get to the goal by the date makes it easy. At first, it may look like hell on earth to you. You might think the idea of actually going through with this to be something on the order of trying to beat a god or something. But, in reality you need to see that if you divide it up in a logical way that it is doable. Any goal that you have is completely doable. You need just to put it in a plan of action and stick to it. By doing it in a daily way, you can chip at it in order to make the huge goal something that you can face.

When you make the daily plan, allow yourself time to put in that goal every day. Going a day without the goal in mind can make things hard on you. You need to leave it there for you to see. If you need to, write it on a sickly note and put it on your fridge. Every single day you'll see that you can reach the goal, and you'll feel motivated to actually work on it and not let it fall by the wayside. You want to have a strong life full of things to do, and putting the goal there each day will get you ready for you to face the hardship of the giant goal.

When you have it all planned out, it's time actually to do it. Even if you think it's one of the worst days ever, you want to have the goal there and work on it. You'll want to dedicate the amount of time that you need to in order to make sure that you reach the goal. It doesn't have to be a lot, but if you make a plan you'll be able to get everything that you need to done. You won't have it hanging around in your head for a long time. You'll also stay on top of things and not let the issues of your laziness take over.

Another thing that you should do is you should always get it done first. It doesn't matter if you need to wake up a tiny bit earlier just to get everything that you need to done for it. Doing it first thing will make things that much better on you. And, if you work on the goal at first, you'll be pumped for the rest of the day. Being pumped and inspired to continue will allow you to continue to make sure that your goals are reached and you're happy.

By doing it first thing and achieving it each day, it also causes morale to be raised. When people are lazy, most of the time they feel like crap. That might be because they don't like just sitting around, but there are other things involved with it as well. You can let you remind wander into places it doesn't need to go when you're sitting around and being idle. It could cause you to think all sorts of weird things, and that's just putting it mildly. By actually making sure that you stay focused, you'll feel better and get more done.

You should also keep yourself motivated. Some days are just draggy and most people hate them. The dog days do happen, and most people hate them. It can be a big issue for so many people, since dog days usually cause people not to want to do anything despite trying. But don't let them get to you. Even if you feel like complete dirt and you just want to sit around and binge-watch Netflix, don't. Don't' do that. Laziness is like a sickness, and if you let that habit in, it'll open up the door for laziness to continue. Instead, keep working on your goals, but also have a plan for what you want to do every single day. Just make up a list of everything that you want to get done, and then just do it. It doesn't take a ton of effort to do so, you just need to have the drive and desire to continue on. It can suck for a while, especially if you're the type who is used to being lax and not doing anything. But, if you knock off the laziness for at least one day, you'll soon realize that at the end of the day, you actually accomplished more than most people. The feeling of accomplishment is remarkable, especially when you accomplish many things. If you keep yourself motivated and want to continue to work, you'll realize later on that doing that could be one of the best things you've ever done for yourself.

Another thing to do in order to help keep time better managed is to get rid of distractions. This one is probably the hardest thing for most people. It's not even the cell phone or the computer. It can be the animals that are making noise, the sound of other appliances, and even the dialogue of people. Distractions are rampant in things, and if they're not taken care of in an effective manner, they can cause a person to get sidetracked easily. Humans are fallible in the fact that they get super sidetracked and off their course easily. One little thing can usually send most people into a tizzy all day. One bad message, or even a good one from a friend, can distract you for god knows how long. You need to realize that these distractions, although nice to have every once in a while, should be eliminated from your life. When people want to talk, just tell them that you're working on something. Some might get offended, but you have to remember that this is your life. You need to make sure that you're getting everything that you need to get done accomplished. It's not that hard, and you have to remember just to keep on going and not care what people think. You're trying to reach your goals, and if a person gets joy out of distracting you from reaching your goal, then they don't deserve to be a friend to you right now. You want to surround yourself with people who support you, and if you need to eliminate them for a bit so you don't' get distracted, it will help you out even more so later on.

A final thing is to reward yourself when you use time effectively. If you get everything that you needed to get done accomplished that day, then that's grounds to celebrate. It's not hard to do, and when you realize it you'll see you've accomplished a big feat. Don't get yourself anything too extravagant until you reach your final goal. Instead, reward yourself a little bit each day whenever you get everything that you need to get done accomplished. You will be happier, and you'll be able to use time to become more efficient as well.

Time efficiency is something everyone struggles with. Everyone seems to have the problem of staying on track and using time wisely. You will be happier, and you'll also reach your goals, which is something that feels amazing.

Chapter 17
Self-Love

The majority of individuals do not think very much about self-improvement. We'd love to assist you in indulging in such a notion and find out just how much you can appreciate yourself. It's a requirement for accepting and creating your ideal weight and everything else that's fantastic for you. Just being conscious of the idea of self-help can move you farther along on the way of enjoying yourself and accepting yourself as possible. Your character is aware of the way you're feeling on your own. If you harbor bitterness or remorse, or sense undeserving, these feelings work contrary to enjoying yourself.

- How can you see your flaws?
- Can you blame yourself? Self-love and finding an error or depriving yourself repaint each other. It is difficult to enjoy yourself if you frequently find errors.
- Can you put attention on negative aspects of yourself?
- Can you end up making self-deprecating statements, such as "I am not intelligent enough to" or even "I am not great enough to..."?
- Can you punish yourself or refuse yourself?
- Can you establish boundaries with individuals who represent your very own moral and ethical criteria and your values and beliefs?

- Look at the mirror. How do you feel about yourself? Can you smile or frown?
- Which are you about the continuum of self?
- Are you currently really respectful and admiring?
- Are you critical and judgmental, or would you love yourself for that you are?
- Have you been caring for this individual who you see?

If you're ambivalent, then contemplate these concerns further. Be truthful with yourself. Have a conversation on your own. Take an honest look at yourself. Do not just examine your own body; examine your wisdom, your soul, and your own emotions, along with your own heart. Know that: By enjoying yourself, you love yourself. When there's something that you can't accept on your own, be aware you could change that idea and alter it to make anything you want, such as your ideal weight.

How does it feel to love yourself?

Have a Look at These characteristics? Are these familiar to you? It is the way it will feel for those who like yourself:

- You genuinely feel happy and accepting your world, even though you might not agree with everything within it.
- You're compassionate with your flaws or less-than-perfect behaviors, understanding that you're capable of improving and changing.
- You mercifully love compliments and feel joyful inside.

- You frankly see your flaws and softly accept them learn to alter them.
- You accept all of the goodness that comes your way.
- You honor the great qualities and the fantastic qualities of everybody around you.
- You look at the mirror and smile (at least all the period).

Many confound self-love with becoming arrogant and greedy. But some individuals are so caught up in themselves they make the tag of being egotistical and thinking just of these. We do not find that as a healthful indulgent, however, as a character that's not well balanced in enjoying love and loving others. It's not selfish to get things your way; however, it's egotistical to insist that everybody else can see them your way too. The Dalai Lama states, "If you do not enjoy yourself, then you can't love other people. You won't have the capacity to appreciate others. If you don't have any empathy on your own, then you aren't capable of developing empathy for others." Dr. Karl Menninger, a psychologist, states it this way: "Self-love isn't opposed to this love of different men and women. You cannot truly enjoy yourself and get yourself a favor with no people a favor, and vice versa." We're referring to the healthiest type of self-indulgent that simplifies the solution to accepting your best good.

Have a better look at the way you see your flaws and blame yourself. Self-love and finding an error or depriving yourself aren't in any way compatible. If you suppress or refuse to enjoy yourself, you're in danger of paying too much focus on your flaws, which is a sort of self-loathing. You Don't Want to place focus on negative aspects of yourself, for holding these ideas in your mind, and You're giving them the psychological energy which brings that result or leaves it actual.

Self-hypnosis can help you use your mind-body to make new and much more loving ideas and beliefs on your own. It helps your mind-body create and take fluctuations in the patterns of feeling and thinking about what has been for you for quite a while, and which aren't helpful for you. The trance work about the sound incorporates many positive suggestions to change your ideas, emotions, and beliefs in alignment with your ideal weight.

An Integral goal for all these positive hypnotic suggestions is the innermost feeling of enjoying yourself. In case your self-loving feelings are constant with your ideal weight, then it is going to occur with increased ease. But if you harbor bitterness or remorse, or sense undeserving, these emotions operate contrary to enjoying yourself enough to think and take your ideal weight. Lucille Ball stated it well: "Love yourself first, and everything falls inline."

The hypnotic suggestions about the sound are directions for change that led to the maximum "internal" degree of mind-body or unconscious. However, the "outer" changes in lifestyle activity should also happen. Many weight-loss approaches you have been using might appear to be a lot of work. We suggest that by adopting a mindset that's without the psychological pressure related to "needing to," "bad or good," or even "simple or hard,"

With no judgment in any way, the fluctuations could be joyous. Yes, joyous.

This produces the whole journey of earning adjustments and shifting easier. The term "a labor of love" implies you enjoy doing this so much, and it isn't labor or responsibility. The "labor" of organizing a family feast in a vacation season, volunteering at a hospital or school, or even buying a present for someone exceptional can appear effortless. Here is the mindset that will assist you in following some weight loss procedures. We invite you to place yourself in the situation of being adored. You're doing so to you. Loving yourself eliminates the job, and that means it is possible to relish your advancement toward a lifestyle that encourages your ideal weight. Think about some action that you like to perform. Imagine yourself performing this action today. Notice that when you're doing something which you like to do, you're feeling energized and enjoyable, and some other attempt is evidenced by enjoyment. What is going on at these times is you "loving what you're doing." Sometimes, we recommend that you also find that as "enjoying yourself doing this." Maybe by directing a more favorable attitude toward enjoying yourself, you'll end up enjoying what you're doing.

Lisa's Brimming Smile

After Lisa and Rick wed, both have been slender and appreciated for their active lifestyles, which included softball and Pilates classes at the local gym. When their very first baby was born, Lisa had obtained an additional fifteen lbs. And now, their second baby came three years after, and she was twenty pounds overweight. Depending on the demands of motherhood, she depended on fast-frozen foods, canned foods, and table food. Persistent sleep deprivation also let her power level reduced, and she can hardly keep up with the toddlers. Rick, a promising young company executive, took more duties on the job, increasing the "ladder of success," indulging in company lunches, and even working late afternoon. He'd return home late, watched the T.V. and eat leftover pizza.

The youthful couple accepted their old way of life but observed with dismay as their bodies grew tired and old beyond their years. However, they lasted. If their oldest boy entered astronomy, they would become more upset. Small Ricky appeared to be the goal of each germfree, and he started to miss several days of college. If this was not enough, he also attracted the germs to the house to his small brother, mother, and father. It appeared that four of these were with them the whole winter.

The infant was colicky. From the spring, following a household bout with influenza, Lisa's friend supplied the title of a behavioral therapist to whom she explained about the ability to shed some light on the recurrent diseases of Lisa's small boys. They were exhausted, tired, not sleeping well, and usually under sunlight. With summer vacation just around the corner, Lisa had been distressed to receive her family back on the right track.

The words of the nutritionist were straightforward: Start feeding yourself along with your household foods, which are fresh and ready in your home. Start buying fruits and veggies, and make some simple recipes using rice and other grains. Learn how to create healthy and wholesome dishes for your loved ones. These phrases triggered Lisa to remember when she had been a kid about the time of her very own small boys. She remembered her mother fixing large fruit salads using lemon. She recalled delicious dishes of homemade soup along with hot fresh bread. Instantly, Lisa knew what she needed to do for her boys. And she'd make it happen. Approximately six months after, we received a telephone call from Lisa. I can hear the grin brimming in her voice. "You cannot think the shift in our loved ones. Ricky has had just one cold in the past six weeks. We are all sleeping much better and also the baby is happy and sleeping during the night. Four days per week, we have a family walk after breakfast or after dinner. And guess what? I have lost thirty-five lbs., and I was not dieting! I'm better than I have ever felt."

Giving Forth

Forgiveness is a significant step in enjoying yourself. At any time, you forgive, you're "committing forth" or "letting go" of a thing you're holding inside you. Let's be clear about this: bias is simply for you, not anybody else. It's not a kind of accepting, condoning, or justifying somebody else's activities. It's a practice of letting go of an adverse impression that has remained within you too long.

It's letting go of any emotion or idea, which can be an obstacle between you and enjoying yourself and getting what you desire.

A lot of us are considerably more crucial and harder on ourselves than we are about others. When you continue to notions of what you need or shouldn't have completed, you aren't enjoying yourself. Instead, you're putting alert energy to negative beliefs about yourself. Ideas like "I must have taken a stroll" or even "I should not have eaten this second slice of pie" can also be regarded as self-punishing. Sometimes, penalizing yourself, either by lack of overeating or eating, may even lead to a discount for your wellbeing. By changing your focus to self-appreciation, you go from the negative to the positive, which is quite a bit more conducive to self-loving.

Writing a diary about all choices you make every day may promote self-improvement.

Chapter 18
Stop Emotional Eating

Understanding the Causes of Emotional Eating

Food choices, while in turmoil, can reflect what emotions are causing your desire to eat. The different types of emotional needs like stress, fatigue, or boredom, prompt you to eat different foods.

Knowing the reason behind emotional eating is the first step to conquering it. Pay attention to how you feel when you eat the foods you eat. You will notice the connection between stress and food.

When you're stressed or frustrated, you tend to look for chewy or crunchy foods like cookies or candy bars. When you're feeling sad, lonely, or depressed, you tend to look for soft or creamy textured foods like ice cream or chocolate. Sadness, loneliness, and depression reflect a lack of love and attention.

When you pay attention to the pattern of eating, you will notice the difference between the two types of eating. Once you identify what is leading you to desire to eat, you can take care of what you need instead of looking for it in food.

This is not the blanket one to identify the connection. It may not work for everyone. There are times you won't identify the specific need that you have but keep searching. Eventually, you will know the exact connection between food and the emotions to a certain degree of accuracy.

Pressure emotions; anger, frustration or resentment

The cravings are for a specific food. You know exactly what you want. The craving is so precise that you can go to the food store to get a specific brand of cookies or nuts. You do what it takes to satisfy the food thought, including getting up in the night to get a bag of French fries.

Foods that you crave when you are frustrated often include nuts, French fries, chewy, meat, hot dogs, pizza or crackers. These foods provide the chewiness or crunchiness that requires an effort to give the feeling of satisfaction. It replaces the thought of having to express the frustration or anger to somebody else. Instead, you direct it to food.

The craving for these foods pops up quickly. Within a minute, you are desperately craving for them. Once you finish eating, you feel better for a while. The food soothes the intense emotions that you had, and you feel calmer and peaceful, albeit temporarily. It is good to note down when this happens so that you can work on it.

Managing Pressure Emotions

When you feel the intense urge to eat chewy or crunchy foods, reflect on what is bothering you. What exactly is irritating or stressing you? Is it that your job is difficult, and you are using food to make it through the day?

Stress, deadlines, and people are a common reason for this eating. When you feel the pressure building, you use food as a quick way to relieve the tension as quickly as possible. Food always seems like the fastest and easiest way than doing yoga or listening to music.

Be honest about how you feel and avoid facing the emotions. Once you identify the cause of how you feel, ask yourself if eating will solve the issue. Will food take away the root cause of the problem?

Will food push over the deadline or remove your stressful boss? If you keep eating, you will get stuck in the same pattern that you desperately want to fix. Eating may seem to solve the problem because you feel better after you eat. But after a few hours, the issue you're running away from will still be there and cause you to eat again. It merely postpones what you should do.

Take the issue heads on and tackle the issue. If it is beyond you, try simple ways to relax like taking a short walk or listen to music. List down activities that you can do on what to do as soon as you start feeling these emotions before your mind shifts the focus to eating.

Keep the list within your reach so that you can retrieve it when you get unexpected emotions. They can be taking a short walk, taking three or more deep breaths, punching on your pillow to release the anger or going to a movie or reading.

When you get a food craving due to these emotions, do just one for the favorite responses that you have selected. Give yourself about ten minutes before you eat anything. These activities may not solve the issue, but they will give your mind time to reflect.

Rather than reaching out for food, think about the root cause of the emotion you're feeling and address it.

Don't fall for the temptation to eat a little bit; you may not manage to stop at one bite.

Feelings of sadness, loneliness, hurt, yearning for love and depression

These feelings make you feel empty, bored, discouraged, depressed, and alone. They don't provoke a specific food craving but push you to eat 'comfort foods.' You wander around the house wanting to eat something, but you don't know what to eat.

You are unsure of what food will feel good for that moment. But you know you want to eat something. When you chose what to eat, you often go for soft and creamy textured foods like ice cream, pies, milkshakes, cake, and pasta. These foods provide a soothing effect and relate to memories of happy times.

The emotions make you yearn to eat what is missing in your life, like love, attention, or appreciation. When emotions come, you eat sweet and smooth foods like cake, ice cream, or sweet foods. Many happy moments are when we eat sweet foods. As a child you probably were comforted with sweet when you cried, so you get hooked to sweets as an adult to recoup the memories where you felt comforted and nurtured.

With these emotions, you don't get instant cravings, but it gradual and vague; making it difficult to identify what is making you desire to eat. You get tempted to use food as a drug to heal your feelings of hurt or loneliness. When ill or tired, you can also be tempted to eat to feel better.

When lonely and anxious, it pushes you to look for something familiar and comforting in food. People eat through all kinds of challenges to get the comfort that food offers. You yearn to get a hug, to be nurtured and comforted. But since you may be all alone, food offers the comfort just temporarily.

Managing These Emotions

Whenever you feel the urge to eat, but you don't know what, reflect on what is happening at that moment. What is prompting your desire to eat? What need do you have? Probably you need a friend, or you have experienced a difficult time, or your life feels boring, and you felt there is something you're lacking.

Ask yourself if eating will change your situation. You may get the short-term soothing and comfort that food provides, but the emotion will still come back if you don't handle the root cause of your feelings. You will still have to deal with the real challenge after the comforting feeling of food wears off. Food temporarily hides the pain, but it doesn't make it disappear.

The best way to handle these emotions is to come up with a list of activities that you can do instead of reaching out for food. The activities include reading, listening to music when you feel sad, or taking a class or a hobby when you feel bored. You can also take a hot shower or soak in the bathtub. Do something nice for yourself like going for manicure or pedicure. Also, consider volunteering at children's home or the elderly home where you can get hugs, and as you comfort others, you will also be comforted. You can also stroke or hold an animal or a stuffed animal.

Most times, you crave a particular food because it reminds you of a time when your needs were met in the past. You eat as a way to recapture the old feelings of happiness prompted by your memory.

Don't wait before everything is perfect before you make changes in your life. You can stop the emotional eating patterns right now and start on a positive way of handling emotions. Any time you feel the urge to eat, ask yourself what the exact issue is. Always remind yourself that food will never solve your problem.

Why We Eat

We should eat to provide our body with nourishment and energy. But we eat for many other reasons. We eat the way we do because of our culture and how we were brought up. We eat out of habit or to satisfy expectations from our peers. Other times we eat in response to our emotions, whether to calm down anger or to comfort us. We also eat from compulsion or as a reward.

The primary reason for eating should be to satisfy the physical hunger, which is the body's way of getting the fuel it needs to function throughout the day. In our current fast-paced society, our intake of food is much greater than we need. Our level of activity is nonexistent. Everything has been made easy to achieve. At work, we labor in our desks until dawn. When we get home, the ease of remote-controlled gadgets keeps us on the couch as we watch TV, dim the lights or close the curtains. The result is that we are suffering from the choices that we have made.

To reverse this, we need to create a life of balance. Plan the day in terms of what activities to do and what food to eat. When there is a sense of balance, you can enjoy life. You balance your nutrition, activities, and rest time. Organize your weekly menu plan and your grocery shopping. Schedule all the activities that you need to do at work and home

The effect of culture on how we eat

Our culture determines our relationship with food. It determines how we combine foods and how we eat food. Some cultures embrace vegetarianism, while others eat more animal meats than plant-based diets. Some cultures place importance on sharing meals and eating together.

The cultural norms play a huge role in the relationship that you have with food. List down some food cultures you can remember growing up so that you can discover the relationship you have with food. List how you can still practice your culture without affecting your relationship with food.

Childhood experiences with food

As adults, we eat just the same way our parents or guardian taught us. Try to remember what food patterns you learned as a child and ho it has impacted your life as an adult.

Some practices include cleaning up your plate. If it was wrong to leave some food on your plate, and you could not leave the dinner table before you finish your food as a child, you will find that as an adult you may overeat so that you don't pour food.

Chapter 19
Portion Control Hypnosis

It can be tempting to give into the promises we see from celebrities and other big brand ads about losing weight. They make it seem so effortless and fun, but when we start the journey ourselves, we soon discover that it is not so simple. This hypnosis is a process that will aide in your weight loss journey and provide for you a natural way to shed the pounds.

You will be guided through the process of feeling better, mindful eating, goal-oriented thoughts, and dedication to the body. This hypnosis is a little different than others and will involve "I" statements. Allow these thoughts to come into your brain as if they were your own.

Natural Weight Loss Hypnosis

Narrator: First you will need to find a calm and quiet place with little distraction. Lay down flat on the ground or bed, or sit with your legs crossed and back comfortably straight, your palms face up and resting on your knees. Once you are in this position begin taking long deep breaths from the stomach, in through the nose, and out the mouth.

Narrator breathes with listener for 5 seconds

Narrator: Good. As you breathe focus in on each of your muscles, letting them constrict and then retract. Move on to the next one.

Constrict, retract. Once all of your muscles are relaxed and your mind has focused on your inner and outer breaths, you'll want to clear your mind of all distractions. Imagine as you exhale, all the worries in your life leave with that one outward breath. Continue this until your mind is completely clear and your breath naturally falls into a rhythm.

Narrator pauses for 3-5 seconds

Narrator: As you continue to focus on these breaths, listen to the words carefully, repeat them in your head if you need to. These are affirmations that will change the way your mind thinks about weight loss and a healthier you. I do not need to participate in any diet plan. I do not need to sign up for one specific workout. I am able to go through with the weight loss all on my own. I am capable and ready to lose the weight naturally, using my own body to do this.

Narrator pauses for 3 seconds

Narrator: My body was designed to keep me as healthy as possible. The first step is deciding that I want to lose weight. This is a step that I have already agreed to. I have continually wanted to lose weight and have this be a part of my lifestyle.

Narrator pauses for 3 seconds

Narrator: I am devoted to making the best decision possible for my health. I am learning self-control and focusing on knowing what the best thing for my body is going to be. I understand when I should say "no," and when I need to push myself through something that might be a bit more challenging. I have recognized what bad habits I have done in the past, and I have created new habits that I can start to add to my future.

Narrator pauses for 3 seconds

Narrator: I understand why I need to lose the weight. I am no longer doing this just for looking good. I am doing this because I need to be healthier. I want to feel good all the time. I want to be able to have confidence and love myself easier.

Narrator pauses for 3 seconds

Narrator: I recognize that I need to love myself in this present moment. I cannot do this journey if I do not believe in myself. I am my own trainer. I am the person that is going to be encouraging me more than anyone else. I am the one who is going to be holding all of the power over my life for the rest of my time on this Earth. I am the one who needs to remember the things that are most important for achieving my dreams.

Narrator pauses for 3 seconds

Narrator: I love myself more than I ever have, which is why I am making this journey. If I do not learn to accept myself the way I am right now, then I will never fully be able to love the person that I am, even after I have made the transformation.

I am my own best friend. I have the ability to lose all of the weight that I want because it is part of who I am. It is natural for me to lose the weight the way that my body designed me to do so.

Narrator pauses for 3 seconds

Narrator: I am going to eat less calories than what I am used to eating right now. I am going to exercise more than what I am used to doing right now. I am going to do this so I can burn more calories and lose even more weight. I am dedicated to this lifestyle because I deserve it. I am focused on shedding the pounds because of all the various health benefits that come along with being more in shape.

Narrator pauses for 3 seconds

Narrator: I am going to eat foods that are healthy for me. I will not deprive myself of any nutrition. I will eat in moderation, but I will never starve myself. I will make sure not to overeat, but I will never completely keep food from my body.

I will exercise as often as I can. I will push myself on days that I feel like staying home instead, but I will never push myself to a point that I physically hurt myself. I will know when I need to try a little harder, and I will know when it is OK to lighten up.

Narrator pauses for 3 seconds

Narrator: I will learn all of these things through trusting my body. Not only do I have the natural processes to lose weight already inside of me, but I have what is needed to trust myself through my own intuition. I understand the importance of listening to my gut.

I recognize how I can read what I need to do, and know what isn't necessary. *Narrator pauses for 3 seconds*

Narrator: I have made mistakes in the past, and there were moments where I didn't judge the situation properly. I will always know how to best listen to my voice as I continue to move forward in this life. I will only grow stronger that voice in the back of my head which tells me what to do. I will listen to my conscious and my subconscious and know how to read both in order to get the truth. I will always be prepared to have to face myself and look deep within my character to get to the root of my issues.

Narrator pauses for 3 seconds

Narrator: I will continue to do this because it is going to help me to lose weight. I will always look for ways to improve the natural methods that I can use to shed the pounds. I am confident in my own abilities to say "no" when it is needed. I won't act on impulse and I will always do my best to control my emotions. The better I can have a handle on my emotions, the easier it will be to know what I need to do to reach my goals and achieve my dreams.

Narrator pauses for 3 seconds

Narrator: I am focused on myself. I am doing this for myself. I am taking care of myself.

Narrator pauses for 3 seconds

Narrator: Each promise that I make to myself is one that brings me closer to my goals. I can feel the air coming in and out of my body.

I am focused on relaxing, because reducing my stress will be important in achieving my goals. I am making a dedication to my body.

Narrator pauses for 3 seconds

Narrator: I am going to provide my body with all of the healthy food, water, air, and sun that it can get. I am like a gorgeous plant that needs the attention it deserves to have a vibrant and healthy blossom. I am devoted to myself. I love myself. I love my body. I am going to take care of my body. I am ready for the future. I am not afraid. I am accepting of the bad. I am excited for what is to come.

Narrator pauses for 3 seconds

Narrator: Take in several deeper breaths, just focusing on your body, your promises, and your goals. As you begin to bring yourself into the conscious, slowly open your eyes, press your palms together at your chest, and smile.

Chapter 20
Additional Tips to Help You Lose Weight

Now, if there's one thing many people are still dealing with in the world today, it's unnecessary weight gain, which is triggered by too much fast food. But with the aid of your side's fitness book, and a few ideas you can try out you will significantly reduce your body's excess fat to give you the youthful look you've had in the past.

While it is a process that takes some time, if you need to get rid of your new body stance at all, you, as the victim, will demonstrate a lot of persistence as well as discipline. And what are some of the tricks with the fitness manual by your side that will make you lose weight within the shortest amount of time? The first thing you can work out is to eat a lot of fruits and vegetables and minimize fat-rich foods.

Having that in mind, you should have a routine follow-up practice that you can do, including taking a short stroll, if you find it challenging to perform rigorous workouts. This will encourage you to eat very balanced foods and do a few light fitness manual exercises from the guidebook.

The other advice is to eat healthy, organic meals, which will contain more vegetables and fruits, and drink green tea after every heart-warming meal you take. This method is very successful, specifically for those who prefer slimming down the natural way. Less calorie intake would also significantly help to decrease the bodyweight because too many calories in the body begin to slow down the body's metabolic process, thereby contributing to the weight already gained.

This is one difficult decision that many people may not be gracious enough to take, but it is the only way out of the weighty issue. Besides, if you choose to consume fewer calorie foods and perform different fitness manual exercises, then your vital body metabolism rate will bounce back into shape faster than you expected. Did you notice that drinking a lot of water will help you lose weight quickly as well?

When you're on a strict diet to lose weight, the body needs to be hydrated all the time to maintain its optimal levels and reduce the excess weight gain and water retention that might be present in the body. You're good to go, with a little fitness boost. Many tips to help you lose weight faster include eating potassium-rich foods, calcium, routine workouts, a healthy diet plan, and a positive attitude throughout.

Forget the anguishing stories you read about how tough it is to lose weight. Make it easier for yourself to help you lose weight by following these ten quick and easy tips. Implement one tip every day, and you'll be at your target weight before you know it: no hassle, and there is no need to turn your whole world upside down either. Don't waste any more time on medications and expensive treatments or hard-earned cash, start to use these tips today and also be lean and healthy.

1. The first trick to help you lose weight is to have healthy eating habits. In this way, you can not only obtain more food quantity, but you can also use natural low-calorie seasonings such as onions to enhance the taste. It is known for long-term wellbeing and weight loss as the diet burden itself is eliminated.

2. Trim the fat always off the meats that you cook. Or if it is chicken-like, cut the fat. Chop it up and add it to something like pasta, if that is too bland!

3. Get a friend accountable for your diet program. People tend to be more committed after a week or two when they know, and need to check in with others. For starters, find someone to walk with, a close friend or even a diet-boyfriend. Say your goals! Sometimes trying to do something by yourself can be a lot harder.

4. To keep track of calories, carbohydrates, proteins, etc., write down everything you consume. You would be shocked if you didn't write down your menu, how many extra items you would drink. Either plan with your dietary intake or start keeping a food log to see!

5. Using a non-stick canola cooking spray, if you need to fry stuff. It will save you plenty of calories over oil cooking. One tablespoon of cooking oil, for example, contains 120 calories! Considering that a 2.4-second PAM spray contains just 16 calories.

6. Keep the outlook optimistic, and never give up. When/if you leave, is the only time you struggle. It may take further work or some other strategy, but it will "will" happen. Studies indicate

that the majority of people struggle to try their first time. Nothing will take the place of determination! Not intellect, not talent, absolutely none! All the rest is secondary.

7. Their diet and wellness programs are 50/50 partners in the weight loss program. When one or the other is missing, you'll have less chance of success! You can work out until you pass out, but you would not see drastic improvements in your appearance if you take too many calories in. And if you don't do exercise, the body is more likely to use muscle rather than fat for energy. Aerobic exercise causes fat burns! Hunger burns up fat!

8. Reflect on the loss of fat and not just the overall weight loss. What matters is your size, and not how much you weigh. You may be surprised because the muscle is more substantial than fat! So know calories burns with the muscle! So eat meals regularly and don't miss it. When you wait for more than four hours, your metabolism will start slowing down.

9. Know where fat appears to get the body. Women seem to accumulate fat around their thighs and glutes. Men gain it on their bellies and around their waist. This is because of the lack of circulation in those regions. Fat isn't taken as quickly into the bloodstream as other regions. That's why fat burning agents such as ephedrine work alongside a long-term weight loss plan. Help even to blood-thinning agents such as aspirin. Still, before using any replacement, make sure you read the labels, directions, and alerts!

10. Keep your weight loss program clear. If you start missing meals or skipping workouts, it slows your progress to the point of

discouragement. How bad do you want that to happen? Select and stick to a good plan. Know, what you put in you gets out of it!

Most people are becoming more conscious of their weight, not just because of how it impacts the way they look but also because of the consequences of their wellbeing. If you're one of those looking to get a leaner body, you certainly should be entertaining the simple but successful techniques.

Turn Your Back on the world of fast food.

Of course, ordering food from a drive-through or over the phone is more relaxed, but if your heart is set to lose significant weight, then this is the first step towards achieving such a goal. You'll have to start eating at home as an option, or if you're a busy person and can't handle such a job, you can always eat at restaurants that have a healthy menu on offer. Turning your back on fast food will also mean giving up processed foods like crispy chips and carbonated drinks.

Apply more liquids to your diet.

Water is a significant factor in the weight loss cycle since it is the carrier of all the nutrients from the food you consume. Keeping this in mind, make sure you drink at least 8 full glasses of water a day, as well as a few glasses of fresh fruit juice. Citrus fruits and berries make excellent shakes because they taste fantastic, and they contain a lot of antioxidants too.

Find the Right Weight Loss Supplement Though – Some people are vehemently opposed to using all kinds of weight loss aids, such as fat-reduction tablets, but having a little boost is nothing wrong. Nonetheless, it is imperative to choose the correct form of supplement and to steer clear of "quick fix items" that are currently very common on the market.

Dedicate 1 hour per day for exercise.

Allot at least one full hour for cardio, no matter how busy you are at home or work. If you have home gym equipment, you can produce quicker results as you can work out daily. An alternative would be to run around your neighborhood block every day for a total of 30 minutes to an hour.

Set Realistic Objectives.

Never expect too much of yourself, and you won't get too upset if your plans don't work out. The best method is to take it one day at a time and let your body adjust to your new diet and exercise routine.

As it's more widely known, celiac disease or Gluten allergy is increasingly becoming more prevalent in the industrialized world in which we reside. Weight gain and celiac disease aren't something that goes hand in hand with weight loss being one of the main factors in Celiac Disease. Have you been diagnosed with Gluten Intolerance lately, and struggled with adding the pounds? Let me give you a few quick tips to add to your diet to help you shed the extra pounds.

I stated above that weight gain, and celiac disease is not generally associated with one another, but that doesn't mean that many people don't have a problem. It's true that almost suddenly, about 99 percent of people will see a dramatic weight loss, and that can have a surprising effect in their daily lives.

Weight gain and suffering from celiac disease. And why do I pour on the pounds?

I'm going to try to explain that quickly and easily. It is essential to know why you could gain weight so you can step on and get rid of the extra weight in your new lifestyle. When you change your diet into Gluten-Free items, many of these don't have the number of nutrients your body wants to perform correctly, and that is an obvious issue. You can get tired, lethargic, and you can feel unwell. No movement or exercise would mean that you don't lose any calories and that you gain weight.

Some of the other causes, and the primary one for many sufferers, is the sudden change in the diet to more high-fat foods. Many people believe it's always low in fat, since a product is gluten-free, and that's not the case. Always read the labels about the products you buy in supermarkets. Many of your local supermarket's pre-packed gluten-free foods might not be as safe as you think, but that does not say that they are not suitable for you. Gluten-free diets are just like any other labeled food; just read the labels first.

Chapter 21
Overcoming Negative Habits

Fortunately, most of our days have a sort of "groove." Actions in a plan that you perform with little thought are performed almost automatically. Otherwise, our lives become tediously complicated, and we spend a lot of time figuring out how to tie our shoes, prepare our meals, go to work, and more. In this way, we can carry out our daily routines with almost no thought and focus our attention on more demanding activities. Repetitive work in life becomes a habit.

Habits can also be undesirable, and these grooves are deeply rooted in today's patterns. They are against us because they waste our time. For example, if you know that you have a limited amount of time to get to work after waking up in the morning, you'll notice that in the middle of breakfast you'll find the morning paper at the table, pick it up, and usually spend the next hour studying. Spend In the daily news, you could spend a good deal of the rest of your time explaining delays or looking for new jobs.

By the way, in our discussion of habits, we call them "desired" or "undesired" rather than "good" or "bad." The words "good" and "bad" have moral implications. These mean certain decisions. In the example cited in the paragraph above, reading a newspaper is not morally "bad," but not desirable at this time.

The terms "desired" and "undesirable" are the terms "ego," meaning self-determination, not decisions made externally. As with psychoanalysis, our goal is to push material from the "conscience" camp into the "ego" realm.

In many cases, you may even say that removing unnecessary habits requires more than a simple choice. You may want to discard your habits consciously, but fulfilling a wish is a very different matter. There are several reasons for this. First, habits are inherent in their definition and are deeply rooted in their behavior, so they are reflected without thinking. Just thinking "I don't do" does not necessarily affect us deep enough to stop unwanted behavior.

The longer the habit we have with us, the more often we do it, the more secure it will be, and the harder it will be to wipe it off. Please quit overeating. It is not uncommon to start eating without knowing it when already taken a full meal or when absorbed in conversation or work. Such behaviors are driven into individual behavioral patterns dozens of times a day, daily, and over ten years, actually becoming a second cortex that is as natural as breathing (ironically, overcoming eating habits are becoming increasingly difficult for people).

Such habits have physical-neurologic-foundation. The neural pathways in our body can be compared to unpaved roads. This road is smooth before vehicles drive on dirt roads. When a car first rides on the road, its tires leave marks, but the ruts are flat. Rain and wind can easily pass by and smooth the road again. However, after 100 rides with deeper and deeper tires, rain and wind make little impression on the deep ruts. They stay there.

The same applies to people. To expand the metaphor a little, we were born with a smooth street in our heads. When a young child first buttons a jacket or ties a shoe, the effort is tedious, clumsy, and frustrating. More trials are needed until the child gets the hang of it, and a successful move becomes a behavioral pattern.

From a physiological point of view, these movement instructions travel along nerve paths to the muscles and back again. The message is sent to the central nervous system along an afferent pathway. The "I want to lift my legs" impulse continues in the efferent pathway from the central nervous system to my muscles: "Raise my legs." After a while, such messages are automatically enriched by countless repetitions and automatically sent at electrical speed.

Return to the car and the street. Suppose the car decides to avoid a worn groove and take a new path. What's going on the car will go straight back into the old ditch. Like people trying to get out of old habits, they tend to revert to old habits.

Still, we haven't developed any unwanted habits. We learn them, and we can rewind the learning. It can be unconditional. And here, self-hypnosis takes place, pushing the individual out of the established habit gap in a smooth manner of new behavior.

The advantage it offers compared to simple willpower trial and error results from an increase in the state of consciousness that characterizes the state of self-hypnosis. A further extension of the unpaved road analogy is that the hovercraft slides a few centimeters above the road, over a rut or habit. Regardless of the habit of working, the implementation process is the same. Only the verbal implant and the image below are different. To encapsulate the induction process, count one, for one thing, two for two things and count three for three things:

1. Please raise your eyes as high as possible.
2. Still staring, slowly close your eyes and take a deep breath.
3. Exhale, relax your eyes, and float your body. Then, if time permits, spend a little more time and introduce yourself to the most comfortable, calm, and pleasant place in your imagination.

Now, when you float deep inside the resting chair, you will feel a little away from your body. It's another matter, so you can give her instructions on how to behave.

At this point, the specific purpose of self-hypnosis determines the expression and image content of the syllogism. It provides suggestions for discussing different habits that can be followed as shown or modified as needed. This strategy can help overcome the habit of overeating.

Overall, we are a country boasting abundant food. Most of us (with the blatant and lamentable exception) have enough money to make sure we are comfortably overeating. As a result, many of us get obese. So, the weight loss business is a big industry. Tablet makers, diet developers, and exercise studios will not confuse customers who want to lose weight.

It is said that every fat person who has a hard time escaping has lost weight. Unfortunately, too often, the lean man spends his life, nevertheless never succeeding in his escape. Despite the image of a funny fat man, everyone rarely enjoys being overweight-most people become unhappy, rarely so confident, and less than confident and ruining their lives. Obesity seems to creep on only some of us, and by the time we notice it, it is a painful habit to overeat or eat, like the excess weight itself.

Self-hypnosis can help this lean man release his bond of "too hard" and start a new life. An article in the International Journal of Clinical and Experimental Hypnosis (January 1975) reports on such cases. Sidney E. and Mitchell P. Pulver cite family doctors study hypnosis in medical and dental practice.

Dr. Roger Bernhardt, while mentioning one of his overweight patients, said that "I brought the patient to the hospital for about a year and a half ago. She went to many doctors to cut back. She said she was rarely leaving home because she was extremely obese; she was relaxing and avoiding people. She came in for £ 380. I started trans in my first session. She continued on a diet and focused on telling her she would like people when she lost weight. She came for the first three or four sessions each week, after which I started teaching her self-hypnosis. Now, this woman lost a total of £ 150, but beyond that, she became another person. She was virtually introverted and rarely came out of her home. She dared to do a part-time job in cosmetics. She hosts a party to show off her cosmetics and hypnotizes herself before the party. She became the state's second-largest saleswoman and earned tens of thousands of dollars."

Simply put, here are the therapies you should use when using self-hypnosis for weight management. After provoking self-hypnosis, mentally recite the syllogism. "I need my body alive. To the extent I want to live, I protect my body just as I protect it."

In the case of a tie mate picture, one can imagine himself in two situations where he is likely to overeat: between meals and at the dining table. With his eyes closed, he imagines a movie screen on the wall. He is on the screen himself, in every situation he finds when he is reading, chatting with others, watching TV, or having trouble calorie counting.

Instead of reaching for popcorn, potato chips, or peanuts as before, he is now simply focusing on the conversation, the television screen, or the printed page, perhaps except for a glass of water, and I congratulate you on being unfamiliar with anything at the table.

The second scene that catches your eye is the dining table. Do you tend to grab this second loaf? Instead, put your hand on your forehead and remember, "Protect my body." Looking at a cake, a loaf, a potato, or a cake raises the idea, "This is for someone. I'm good enough". With the fork down, take a deep breath and be proud to help one-person flow through the body.

Then, imagine a very simple and effective exercise method that simply puts your hand on the edge of the table and pushes it. Better yet, stand up from the chair and leave the table at this point.

Here's another image I'd recommend to a self-hypnotist. If you introduce yourself to the screen of this fictional movie, you will find yourself slim. Give yourself the ideal line that you want to see to others. Cut the abdomen and waistline to the desired ratio. Take an imaginary black pencil, sketch the entire picture, and make the lines sharp and solid. Hold photo because you can keep this slender picture, you can lose weight.

Then get out of your hypnosis and repeat it regularly every few hours. Exercise is especially useful during the temptation to be used as a comfortable, calorie-free substitute for fatty snacks or as an additional serving with meals. It would be a good time to practice it just before dinner.

Chapter 22
Mistakes to Avoid

Are you ready to begin your journey to intuitive eating? The process is straight forward but takes some practice to adapt to your body and needs. Set goals for yourself: learn to read your body's signals and communication.

Avoid Skipping Meals

This is good advice for anyone. Skipping meals is sometimes inevitable, especially if your schedule doesn't allow much time to take a break. If you expect this to happen and can prepare ahead, get up early to start breakfast early. Pay attention to your level of hunger in the morning, to determine how much you want to eat. Bring a light snack to work or school, just in case there is an opportunity to satisfy your hunger, should you feel this way and need to prolong or skip lunch. Whether you eat small or large meals, ensure that you have something nutritious and tasty, just in case. Even the best-planned schedules can change at the last minute and being prepared can alleviate a lot of unnecessary stress.

Not Drinking Enough Water

Hunger can be a symptom of dehydration. If you feel hungry, drink water first. Being hydrated is one of the most important ways to stay healthy. It can also regulate your hunger signals so that when you feel like eating, it is a response to hunger and not for other reasons. If drinking water during the day doesn't appeal to you, try adding lemon, lime or cucumber. Sparkling water can be another alternative. Herbal teas are great during colder months, to ensure you are hydrated. Fruit contains a lot of water and natural sugar, which can provide a boost in energy in between meals if needed. Coffee is acceptable in moderation, though alternate drinking coffee with water, as it can have a dehydrating effect.

Setting Unrealistic Goals

Many of us set goals when we diet, and often, they can be unrealistic. Magazines, advertisements and diet programs promote quick fixes and sure-fire ways to lose weight fast, but this is only good in the interim. In extreme cases, where weight loss is necessary for health reasons, a medical professional or nutritionist may provide a specific guideline for eating. Even within this plan, mindful eating can be practiced, by noticing how the food you eat impacts you and when you eat. Choosing healthy foods can be counterproductive if we eat when we're not hungry or too much when we are, therefore not listening to our signals.

Focus on one goal at a time, if necessary, to avoid discouragement and disappointment. In other words, don't expect to lose a lot of weight, reduce your anxiety and lower your sugar levels all at once, though if you eat relatively healthy and exercise, even moderately, you'll likely see positive results within a few weeks. The key is not to expect overnight transformations that you can post on social media for a shocking response. Even the most successful people, when it comes to losing one hundred pounds or becoming athletic, must dedicate months, even years, to achieving their goals. When the goal is reached, maintenance is still needed and must continue. Mindfulness can instill that level of maintenance from the very beginning so that it becomes part of your everyday way of living.

Obstacles to Intuitive Eating: Emotional Response to Food and Changing Habits

We all have habits that are difficult to break or change, and it's not something that can be achieved overnight. Recognizing a negative habit is a start to making an improvement, as it shows we are aware of it. Habit forming traits often happen as a response to something else in our life. For example, we may overeat when we feel emotionally upset or as a way to make ourselves feel better when we have a challenging experience. This can happen when someone is grieving or feeling a sense of loss. Food can often take the place of that loss in order to cope. When you are going through a difficult time, it's important to not blame yourself, especially for eating habits. Realize that it is temporary, and in time, when you are ready, you can change the way you think about eating. The key is awareness. A helpful approach is a meditation, to give yourself that space to reflect, without judgment, and set realistic goals.

Avoid Multi-Tasking When You Eat

Meeting a deadline, chatting online or in person, and getting work done are all activities that many people try to accomplish during a meal. This happens most often during lunch break, as a "working lunch" or as a way to save time and alleviate the stress of having to complete the work after lunch, though the opposite will occur. As you try managing both tasks, you're eating habits and connecting with your body's signals will interfere. This breaks the connection between your food and you. It is during this multi-tasking that you may feel more anxious to rush back to work from lunch, or in a more social and conversational atmosphere, lose that sensation you experience when you enjoy your meal alone and without distraction. Even if you are pressed for time, leaving a minimum of twenty minutes to enjoy a meal is a good start. Put down the files, leave the computer screen and go for a walk in a quiet and serene place. Meals, whenever you choose to enjoy them and when you can find adequate time and space for them, should take center stage, and all other events put on pause until you are finished.

If you enjoy eating with coworkers, family, and friends, make it an enjoyable event. Keep it positive and fun. If a working lunch is what you want to do, find that enjoyment in your food when you can and chew, savor every mouthful. Keep multi-tasking to a minimum, if you have to keep tasks in motion during your break. Your team may notice how you slow down to eat and enjoy the taste of your food. It may be appropriate to talk about the food and appreciate what you have. This may encourage others to see how you approach intuitive eating and could motivate them as well!

Chapter 23
The Importance of Habits

Behind every habit, there is a real need that you need to satisfy. Be it any kind of habit, good or bad. Like for example:

- Who smokes to relieve stress?

- Who drinks to relax?

- Whoever exercises for pleasure?

All of these activities, whether harmful or not, contain a yearning for fulfillment for those who practice. This is what makes a habit so difficult to change.

So much so that when trying to change a habit, you will experience great difficulty in the first few weeks.

Because, when you stop doing something that was already customary, your body will begin to crave that sensation caused by that old custom that you left behind.

Tips to improve your habits

Life is full of habits, good and bad, it is just as easy to have positive habits as negative, but transforming them implies an effort and a lot of willpower, a change of beliefs and appreciation.

The answer is in you, can you change your habits?

- Know the habits you would like to adopt. Start by making a detailed list of the habits you would like to change or improve.

- Analyze the attitudes that general conflicts. If you have not been able to identify all the bad habits or do not think you do not have them, ask yourself what kind of behaviors generate conflicts in your daily life and with the people around you, an example would be if you arrive at your appointments late and this causes discomfort in other people if you have no energy because you do not eat healthily or if you are a little overweight and you dislike it.

- Become aware of the importance of changing bad habits. It is important to raise awareness in a subtle way, to the people closest to you about the importance of improving their habits. If they do it simultaneously, it will be easier to adopt them. For example, if someone in your family buys junk food and you are looking for a healthy diet, it is important to encourage them not to do so so that everyone improves their habits and their diet, especially if this person is overweight.

- Build an action plan. Once you have identified the habits you would like to adopt, you need to make an action plan to carry it out. The first step is to become aware of the habit you want to change and constantly monitor your actions and thinking patterns to identify why you react that way. The next thing will be to repeat the new habit every day for at least 30 days, and it is the minimum time in which a habit is adopted. For example, if you want to start exercising, do it at least four days a week for two months. In this way, your body and mind will adapt to the new activities you do.

- Be honest with yourself. Finally, it is necessary that you be objective and recognize if you have continued repeating the new habits, analyze if you already feel that they are part of your daily life. If not, it is important to analyze the causes that prevented you from achieving it.

Habits are nothing more than the daily repetition of an attitude and discipline. The best day to start changing your habits is today. If you stop to think about all the time it takes to change a habit, and you probably won't, the important thing is to be determined and start today.

How to Improve Your Eating Habits for Weight Loss

The barriers people have reached for they seem to have no end in sight. Hunger, fruit diets and uncooked foods are among the drastic alternatives to the long old weight-loss problem. I had made an attempt to try these for myself, and none of them succeeded until I closed the diet and only changed my weight loss eating habits.

The diets are similar to weight loss band-aids. In a short-term illness, they are a fast solution and do not change behavior, metabolism or produce a true bang on body fat. Dietary rigidity does not increase the element of success; in reality, it decreases it. It is much easier to make gradual changes that are not upsetting or penalizing but launch the body on the road to equilibrium and its normal set point to some extent. Stable changes in eating habits are certainly a great option for losing weight.

Rather than eliminating calories by the end of the day or for a big meal, five or six small food portions are much healthier for the body. This sounds contradictory, but real. The body burns calories in everyday exercise. This requires food calories to feed and digest. Reports show that up to 10% of calories are used to process the food.

Therefore, 50 calories are needed for food processing for a 500-calorie serving. It's been shown that eating less often helps in weight gain over the long term. To strengthen your weight-loss eating habits, you will regularly consume yet healthy foods. A psychosomatic eating benefit is feeling good. The feeling you're not hollow is beneficial in continuing the weight loss cycle.

Booming weight loss isn't a major science, nor does it entail difficulty and pain. Easy changes like cooking nutritious meals 5-6 times a day. Eating the right part size is critical. Eating the right calories is important, and daily exercise is important. Eat and consume the right form of food are the safest dietary habits for weight loss. If you follow this advice, I'm sure the pounds will go smoothly.

Eating Habits for Weight Loss

- Feed gradually-At 100 mph too many of us are guilty of feeding. We have to slow down our feeding, really. A good way to look at it is that the quicker we eat, the more we consume, the more we consume, the more money we spend!! As a guideline, aim to start eating at 1/4 of your current pace, and you can add the pennies as you drop the pounds!!

- Wait 20 minutes after each meal-How many times have you reached directly for the biscuit tin or for some ice cream thinking that you're not yet full? It takes about 20 minutes for the message to hit our brain once we are complete. Therefore, we are free to continue eating as much as we want within that 20 minutes (or until our stomach can hold no more), even though we have already eaten enough to meet the needs of our bodies.

- Avoid distractions when eating-this may be difficult, but who is guilty of eating on the TV, the Internet, a magazine, a friend's phone, etc.? Think back to a time when you demolished a big box of sweet popcorn without even taking your eyes from the screen? Yeah, where did anything go? Unconsciously, eating can lead to severe unhealthy food, so take the time to sit at the dinner table and take care of what you consume.

Chapter 24
Frequently Asked Questions

Can I use hypnosis to lose weight?

Weight loss hypnosis can help you lose excess weight if it is part of a weight loss plan that includes diet, exercise, and counseling. ... Hypnosis is usually done with the help of a hypnotherapist using repeated words and spiritual images.

How Well Does Hypnosis Work For Weight Loss?

For those who want to lose weight, hypnosis may be more effective than just eating and exercising. The idea is that it can affect the mind to change habits like overeating. ... The researchers concluded that hypnosis may promote weight loss, but there is not enough research to convince it.

Is Hypnosis Dangerous?

Hypnosis performed by a trained therapist or medical professional is considered a safe and complementary alternative. However, hypnosis may not be appropriate for people with severe mental illness. The side effects of hypnosis are rare, but may include the following:

Can Hypnosis Change Your Personality?

No, hypnosis doesn't really work at all. But that is a fun premise. That said, hypnosis helps with stress, bad (and good) habits, sleep deprivation and quality, and pain management. ... In that case, no, hypnosis cannot change personality.

How can I Tell If Someone Is Hypnotized?

The following changes do not always occur in all hypnotic subjects, but most are seen sometime during the trance experience.

- Stare. ...
- Pupil dilation. ...
- Change in blinking reflection. ...
- Rapid eye movement. ...
- The eyelids flutter. ...
- Smoothing facial muscles. ...
- Breathing slows down. ...
- Reduced swallowing reflex.

How Long Does It Take For Hypnosis To Work?

Depending on what the client's goal is, the client will appear on average between 4-12 sessions. Imagine for some time that you are my client and that you are sitting in my comfortable "hypnotic chair".

What Are The Negative Effects Of Hypnosis?

There are several risks associated with hypnosis. The most dangerous is the possibility of creating incorrect memories (called confabulations). Other potential side effects include headache, dizziness, and anxiety. But these usually disappear immediately after the hypnosis session.

What Is The Hypnosis Success Rate?

The study found that hypnosis had long-term changes in an average of six hypnosis sessions, while psychoanalysis took 600 times. In addition, hypnosis was very effective. After 6 sessions, 93% of participants had a recovery rate of only 38% in the psychoanalysis group.

Does Hypnosis Work When I Sleep?

Hypnosis is not sleep (a meditation with a goal), but if you are tired, you can fall asleep while listening to hypnosis. ... Fortunately, hypnosis reaches the subconscious even if it falls asleep.

How Much Weight Can I Lose With Hypnosis?

Most studies show a slight weight loss, with an average loss of about 6 pounds (2.7 kilograms) over 18 months. However, the quality of some of these studies has been questioned and it is difficult to determine the true effectiveness of weight loss hypnosis.

Does Meditation Lose Weight?

Although there isn't a lot of research that shows that meditation can directly help you lose weight, meditation can help you better understand your thoughts and actions, including those related to food.

Can Everyone Be Hypnotized?

If we understand hypnosis as a focused state of attention, where there is not necessarily a loss of consciousness or lack of memory about what has happened in the session, the answer is yes. But if we understand this question as if the whole world can reach deep trance (sleepwalking) - understood in terms of classical hypnosis - with practically total suggestibility and loss of consciousness, the answer would be a relative NO.

Getting a light or medium trance is relatively easy. Reaching a deep trance is more complex; approximately 80% of subjects can reach a deep stage without much difficulty. The remaining 20% would be difficult due to several complicated variables of knowing or controlling (fear of losing one's conscience, prejudices or beliefs, lack of confidence in the inducer, etc.) Despite this fact, if we use hypnosis at the clinical level or doctor, in most cases a medium trance is enough to obtain results 2. - Who can hypnotize?

Hypnosis is essentially a technique. Therefore, anyone who knows it enough and learns to apply it can hypnotize. Another thing is that the inductor can then confront and solve the different situations that arise during the session. If the hypnotist does not have concrete and sufficient theoretical-practical knowledge (even if they are doctors or psychologists), it could cause serious damage to the hypnotist. Even more so if the inducer pursues unlawful ends and tries to violate the physical, psychic or moral integrity of the inducer, which has happened numerous times, manipulating the hypnotized.

Can Someone Fall Asleep Forever?

It is completely impossible for it to happen. Whether we practice self-hypnosis (about ourselves), or hetero-hypnosis, that is, about another person, we will always end up leaving the hypnotic state. If for any reason the hypnotist disappeared, the induced subject would progressively move from the hypnotic trance to natural sleep and would gradually wake up and clear. It happens sometimes that the person is in such a placid situation that he resists waking up. In that case we can make a counter-suggestion such as: "If you want to stay or return to this state in the future, you must wake up now" - and will normally abandon hypnosis. Or we just let it rest until it wakes up after a time that is usually short.

Does Hypnosis Have Contraindications?

Hypnosis and all similar states and techniques produce a great benefit to the organism, since it helps eliminate physical or emotional tensions, slightly reduces blood pressure, regulates the heart and respiratory rhythm, balances the cerebral hemispheres and if we talk in energetic terms, rebalances the body's bioenergy. Therefore, if we are normally healthy people, we will not be in any danger.

However, there are two absolute indications: in general, hypnosis should not be performed on people with schizophrenia or serious mental illness. Why? Because we could aggravate their symptoms apart from that they would be difficult to induce. The second case is about people with epilepsy or who have had recent crises of this type: during hypnosis one of these crises could occur, so prudence advises not to submit them. 5. - Does the hypnotist have any special power?

Strongly NO. When hypnosis is used as a show, the hypnotist usually presents himself with an aura of exceptional mental powers; this is part of the suggestive environment that the inductor will use to achieve its spectacular effects. It all depends on how suggestible and impressionable we are.

Really if a person does not want it, it is very difficult to be induced, unless there is such an extreme fear or conviction that the hypnotist has such (fictitious) power that our own belief or conviction will make us fall into hypnosis even sometimes instantaneously to the slightest suggestion or touch of the inductor. To hypnotize you do not need special skills, but a minimum of skills. For example, a shy, doubtful and insecure person would be a bad hypnotist or hypnotist.

Can Someone Be Induced To Do What They Do Not Want?

Although several authors deny this possibility, our practice only for experimental purposes shows us that YES. Everything depends on many different variables, but if the induced subject has a sufficient degree of hypnotic depth, he can accept, in whole or in part, the possibility of refusing the suggestions imposed by the hypnotist. There have been numerous cases of rape and mental manipulation under states of hypnosis - this is nothing new - That is why we should not be hypnotized by people who do not have our confidence.

Can We Hypnotized Ourselves?

Of course. Self-hypnosis is one of the most interesting aspects of this technique. For this we can use - for example - a cassette, where we will record an induction to relax progressively, including suggestions such as: "I am getting calmer, my muscles are released, little by little I feel a pleasant and deep reverie ... "In the end, we will add the suggestions that we want to implement for various purposes, such as studying more and better, quitting tobacco, being calmer, etc.

Can You Hypnotize Us Without Us Noticing?

Hypnosis is more present in our lives than we imagine. In fact, if this is only a state of attention more or less acute and focused, every day we suffer to a greater or lesser extent one or more "hypnosis." Advertising - especially on TV aims to hypnotize us (suggest us) to buy a product ... politicians use very elaborate communication and image techniques to capture our attention, even where the final impression is more important than the speech itself. But returning to classical hypnosis, there are subliminal techniques to induce a subject to hypnotic states and induce him, without the need for loss of consciousness - to certain behavior or attitude.

Is There Instant Hypnosis?

Yes. For example in hypnotic shows, when the inductor realizes that someone among his audience is very suggestible and even shows some fear when approaching him, his own fear and the fact that the hypnotist is seen wearing a special power, will make the slightest hint of it, the viewer immediately falls into hypnosis (normally it will be a light or medium trance and will have to be deepened).

The other case would be when once an induction is achieved, the subject is left implanted with a post-hypnotic order such as: "when you wake up and on the next occasions when I tell you, you will immediately fall into this same state" If the achieved state is deep enough, it is implanted in the subject's deep mind and can last even for an indefinite period.

Can You Hypnotize From A Distance?

This is one of the most Apasio Nantes research fields in the field. It is disturbing to see that in many occasions under hypnosis mental activity, its scope and scope of knowledge will exceed space and time. Our nervous system is a true network through which low voltage electricity circulates; where there is electricity, electro-magnetism can be given, so that the network of extended neurons throughout our anatomy becomes a virtual frequency transmitter that can incorporate certain information.

Chapter 25
Create Reasonable Goals

Manage Your Expectations

It's good to want to push yourself to be the best that you can be and strive to be a brand-new person. Having huge expectations for yourself can help you create and achieve your goals. It's healthy to believe in your power to have enormous success. It's okay to want dramatic changes, but keep in mind that you need to be realistic with yourself. Take this process day by day if you have to, but know that you will get results eventually, but how long and how much those results require will vary based on what you experience along that journey and how well you respond to hypnotherapy. Everyone will react to these changes differently, and it doesn't make anyone better or worse than anyone else.

It's okay to take it slow. Work at your own pace and be fine with the pace that you are working at. Don't compare how fast you are losing weight to how fast other people are losing weight. Some people may be able to lose two or even three pounds in a week while you may struggle just to lose one. That doesn't mean you're not doing well. Comparison can be deadly for diets, so focus on your own progress instead of desperately trying to keep up with other people. Your body is unique, and your pace is all your own. Take pride in your pace, no matter what that pace is because any progress is better than what most people accomplish, so that's something to celebrate!

Because repetition helps people absorb information, I'm going to reiterate once more that you shouldn't expect instantaneous changes. This is going to be a lifetime pursuit. This is not a diet that has a beginning and an end. We are programmed to believe that weight loss routines have an expiration date, and for that reason, diets often fail. An end date suggests that you can go back to how you were before. The point of this is not to return to the person you used to be. The point of the changes I endorse is to make it so that you don't want to go back to behaving how you used to behave. Hypnosis allows you to make changes and normalizes them to your brain so that those changes become habitual, and you're able to do them consistently.

Be aware of your body's limits. Some people just aren't going to be able to start running miles at a time. Some people will never be able to do that. Your body has limits, and there's nothing wrong with having limits. You can expand upon your limits, but make sure you don't push yourself too far, too soon. If you hurt your health or injure yourself, you're going to have more trouble staying active and eating right, so take care of your body. It's the only one you have, and if you neglect its needs and push it more than it can handle, you're not being reasonable with yourself.

Don't force yourself to do things that only feel like a chore. You need to create expectations that will make your life not just bearable but pleasurable. Most importantly, stop grumbling about the changes you need to make. They are hard, but negativity only creates more negativity. If you can find the positives, you will feel better about your entire situation and be able to keep up with all the plans that you have made. If you ever start dragging your feet during this process, make some changes that put some pep in your step.

Be flexible. Any plan worth having should have enough wiggle room that you can take detours on the way without your whole plan being derailed. Like you need to be open to the changes, you need to be open to how you'll have to adjust what you are doing based on your circumstances. Weight loss takes months or even years, so your needs now may not meet your needs in the future. If you get sick, for example, you may have to put exercise on pause and shift your diet for a while. This is just a bump in the road, and if you're flexible, you can endure it.

Lots of bumps in the road may make you feel disheartened. Be prepared for obstacles. They're going to happen. Lots of them. You'll have bad days that make you feel like you'll never get back on track. You'll overeat sometimes, and you'll fall off track with your exercise regime. Sometimes, you'll just feel bad. You'll be upset about your lack of progress. You'll be desperate to hurry up and get the weight off already. Tragedies, like a death in the family, may impact your emotions and make it harder to keep true to your diet, but these obstacles are all part of life, and learning to handle them and your weight at the same time is how you create lifelong change.

Be merciful with yourself. Don't be too harsh on yourself for mistakes or the way you handle the obstacles you face because you probably wouldn't be that harsh with anyone else. If you wouldn't be as hard on your best friend as you're being on yourself, you need to be gentler with yourself. Treat yourself as you would treat the people who are most dear to you. Practice positive self-talk and expect that the people in your life talk positively about you as well.

Don't expect magic. Even with hypnosis, you're going to have to put in a lot of work. If it starts to feel too easy, push yourself a little more. Don't let yourself get complacent with your weight loss. Continue to push your mind and body towards where you want them to go. Your expectations will outline your progress. Maintain your expectations for yourself because expectations are what will show you whether you've made progress or not. Always keep your expectations in mind so that you can remind yourself of what you want and why you want it. Celebrate your progress as it happens, and the weight loss will feel magical just because of how good it makes you feel.

Good Goals Are Hard to Find

Goals help you get where you want to go better than anything else. You need them to navigate the curves of life. If you want to get anywhere in life, it helps to have a clear plan of where you want to go. If you get in the car and drive aimlessly, it's going to be a lot harder to find the destination you are yearning to find. Hypnosis is hard if you don't know what you want; however, if you know where you'd like to be, suddenly, hypnosis becomes like a GPS. All you have to do is enter where you'd like to go, and your hypnotist will guide you to the location. You'll still have complete control of the car, and only your goals will guide the session.

Making goals is a big deal because most people fail to make goals at all, which is detrimental to their progress. A Harvard Business study showed that only fourteen percent of people even make goals. Further, those with goals are ten times more successful at accomplishing what they want to accomplish than those who do not make goals. Thus, the feat of simply making goals is a huge step that brings you just a little bit closer to making your aspirations come true. Accordingly, be clear with yourself about what you want so that you know exactly what to work towards.

Make incremental goals. Incremental goals help you from feeling overwhelmed. When you're overwhelmed, you shut down and become unable to make any progress. Thus, don't let yourself get overwhelmed by making a series of small goals to build up to your bigger goal. Use these goals to propel yourself forward. Incremental goals serve as mile markers that mark the progress you've made. You can celebrate those little victories and use them as motivation to keep going. Always keep the larger goal in your mind but focus on the smaller goals as you get to them.

Your goals should make you feel energized, and they should be measurable. A goal of "being the weight that makes me happy," isn't going to give you much direction and will do little to push you forward. When your goals are too abstract or vague, they will quickly lose steam, and you won't have the energy to complete them. Be sure to have ways to quantify your goals so that you can see how much closer you are to your objective. Your goals should excite you throughout your journey and make you excited to complete them. If that motivation is ever lost, you need to reevaluate.

The quality of your goals matter. Be clear about what you want. Don't make half-hearted goals. Half-hearted goals aren't going to satisfy you, and they aren't going to give you any direction, either, making them useless. Even if your goal is measurable, if it is not achievable or won't challenge you at all, it is not a quality goal. Find goals that you can invest fully in. Find goals that make you motivated to work hard for a long time to come.

No matter what your goals are, write your goals down. Only three percent of people make written goals, but those people are three times as successful as those who have goals but have not written them. This statistic shows how powerful it is to write your goals down. By writing them down, your declaring your dedication to those goals, and you feel more motivated to keep up that goal when it's preserved on a piece of paper. When you write something down, you commit to it, and you feel accountable for that objective you've written down.

Create a timeline for your goals. By January 15, a whopping ninety-two percent of New Year's resolutions have been discarded, which shows how quickly people can throw their goals aside until another year rolls around. Thus, creating a timeline for when you want to accomplish which goals can help keep you on track. While having deadlines for a certain amount, you want to lose can be helpful, don't become too rigid with your timeframe. If you can't keep up with what you thought you could do, adjust your plan instead of falling terribly behind and quitting. Allow yourself to adapt to how your body reacts to dieting so that you never lose sight of what you want while still being open-minded.

Allow your goals to change over time. What you want out of hypnosis, and your weight loss journey may change over time, which is why you should be ready to change your goals when your interests shift. Goals should give you the drive you need to complete them, but if they don't, that's a clear indicator that you need to reevaluate what is motivating you and find new motivators.

Chapter 26
Learn to Avoid Temptations and Triggers

While telling a person to adopt the traits of the mentally strong is a good way to develop mental toughness, it may not always be enough. In a way it's a bit like telling a person that in order to be healthy you need to eat right, exercise, and get plenty of rest. Such advice is good and even correct, however it lacks a certain specificity that can leave a person feeling unsure of exactly what to do. Fortunately, there are several practices that can create a clear plan of how to achieve mental toughness. These practices are like the actual recipes and exercises needed in order to eat right and get plenty of exercise. By adopting these practices into your daily routine, you will begin to develop mental toughness in everything you do and, in every environment, you find yourself in.

Keep your emotions in check

The most important thing you can do in the quest for developing mental toughness is to keep your emotions in check. People who fail to take control of their emotions allow their emotions to control them. More often than not, this takes the form of people who are driven by rage, fear, or both. Whenever a person allows their emotions to control them, they allow their emotions to control their decisions, words, and actions. However, when you keep your emotions in check, you take control of your decisions, words, and actions, thereby taking control of your life overall.

In order to keep your emotions in check you have to learn to allow your emotions to subside before reacting to a situation. Therefore, instead of speaking when you are angry, or making a decision when you are frustrated, take a few minutes to allow your emotions to settle down. Take a moment to simply sit down, breathe deeply, and allow your energies to restore balance. Only when you feel calm and in control should you make your decision, speak your mind, or take any action.

Practice detachment

Another critical element for mental toughness is what is known as detachment. This is when you remove yourself emotionally from the particular situation that is going on around you. Even if the situation affects you directly, remaining detached is a very positive thing. The biggest benefit of detachment is that it prevents an emotional response to the situation at hand. This is particularly helpful when things are not going according to plan.

Practicing detachment requires a great deal of effort at first. After all, most people are programmed to feel emotionally attached to the events going on around them at any given time. One of the best ways to practice detachment is to tell yourself that the situation isn't permanent. What causes a person to feel fear and frustration when faced with a negative situation is that they feel the situation is permanent. When you realize that even the worst events are temporary, you avoid the negative emotional response they can create.

Another way to become detached is to determine the reason you feel attached to the situation in the first place. In the case that someone is saying or doing something to hurt your feelings understand that their words and actions are a reflection of them, not you. As long as you don't feed into their negativity you won't experience the pain they are trying to cause. This is true for anything you experience. By not feeding a negative situation or event with negative emotions you prevent that situation from connecting to you. This allows you to exist within a negative event without being affected by it.

Accept what is beyond your control

Acceptance is one of the cornerstones of mental toughness. This can take the form of accepting yourself for who you are and accepting others for who they are, but it can also take the form of accepting what is beyond your control. When you learn to accept the things you can't change, you rewrite how your mind reacts to every situation you encounter. The fact of the matter is that the majority of stress and anxiety felt by the average person is the result of not being able to change certain things. Once you learn to accept those things you can't change, you eliminate all of that harmful stress and anxiety permanently.

While accepting what is beyond your control will take a little practice, it is actually quite easy in nature. The trick is to simply ask yourself if you can do anything at all to change the situation at hand. If the answer is 'no,' simply let it go. Rather than wasting time and energy fretting about what you can't control adopt the mantra "It is what it is." This might seem careless at first, but after a while you will realize that it is a true sign of mental strength. By accepting what is beyond your control, you conserve your energy, thoughts, and time for those things you can affect, thereby making your efforts more effective and worthwhile.

Always be prepared

Another way to build mental toughness is always to be prepared. If you allow life to take you from one event to another you will feel lost, uncertain, and unprepared for the experiences you encounter. However, when you take the time to prepare yourself for what lies ahead, you will develop a sense of being in control of your situation at all times. There are two ways to be prepared, and they are equally important for developing mental toughness.

The first way to be prepared is to prepare your mind at the beginning of each and every day. This takes the form of you taking time in the morning to focus your mind on who you are, what you are capable of, and your outlook on life in general. Whether you refer to this time as mediation, contemplation, or daily affirmations, the basic principle is the same. You simply focus your mind on what you believe and the qualities you aspire to. This will keep you grounded in your ideals throughout the day, helping you to make the right choices regardless of what life throws your way.

The second way to always be prepared is to take the time to prepare yourself for the situation at hand. If you have to give a presentation, make sure to give yourself plenty of time to prepare for it. Go over the information you want to present, choose the materials you want to use, and even take the time to make sure you have the exact clothes you want to wear. When you go into a situation fully prepared, you increase your self-confidence, giving you an added edge. Additionally, you will eliminate the stress and anxiety that results from feeling unprepared.

Take the time to embrace success

One of the problems many negatively-minded people experience is that they never take the time to appreciate success when it comes their way. Sometimes they are too afraid of jinxing that success actually to recognize it. Most of the time, however, they are unable to embrace success because their mindset is simply too negative for such a positive action. Mentally strong people, by contrast, always take the time to embrace the successes that come their way. This serves to build their sense of confidence as well as their feeling of satisfaction with how things are going.

Next time you experience a success of any kind, make sure you take a moment to recognize it. You can make an external statement, such as going out for drinks, treating yourself to a nice lunch, or some similar expression of gratitude. Alternatively, you can simply take a quiet moment to reflect on the success and all the effort that went into making it happen. There is no right or wrong way to embrace success, you just need to find a way that works for you. The trick to embracing success is in not letting it go to your head. Rather than praising your efforts or actions, appreciate the fact that things went well. Also, be sure to appreciate those whose help contributed to your success.

Be happy with what you have

Contentment is another element that is critical for mental toughness. In order to develop contentment, you have to learn how to be happy with what you have. This doesn't mean that you eliminate ambition or the desire to achieve greater success, rather it means that you show gratitude for the positives that currently exist. After all, the only way you will be able to appreciate the fulfillment of your dreams truly is if you can first appreciate your life the way it is.

One example of this is learning to appreciate your job. This is true whether you like your job or not. Even if you hate your job and desperately want to find another one, always take the time to appreciate the fact that you have a job in the first place. The fact is that you could be jobless, which would create all sorts of problems in your life. So, even if you hate your job, learn to appreciate it for what it is. This goes for everything in your life. No matter how good or bad a thing is, always appreciate having it before striving to make a change.

Be happy with who you are

In addition to appreciating what you have you should always be happy with who you are. Again, this doesn't mean that you should settle for who you are and not try to improve your life, rather it means that you should learn to appreciate who you are at every moment. There will always be issues that you want to fix in your life, and things you know you could do better. The problem is that if you focus on the things that are wrong you will always see yourself in a negative light. However, when you learn to appreciate the good parts of your personality, you can pursue self-improvement with a sense of pride, hope, and optimism for who you will become as you begin to fulfill your true potential.

Chapter 27
How to Build Motivation

Motivation is one of the most powerful tools in creating permanent change. Your motivation is based on what you believe. And as you are probably aware, belief is scarcely based on your concrete reality. In essence, you believe things because of how you see them, feel them, hear them, smell them, and so forth. You can program your mind by taking feelings from one of your experiences and connecting those feelings to a different experience. Let us look at how you can remain motivated to lose weight:

Establish Where You Are Now

You should take a full-length picture of yourself at the present as a push mechanism from your current position, as well as for comparison later on. Two primary factors are relevant to health. One is whether you like the image you see in the mirror and the second is how you feel. Do you have the energy to do what you wish, and are you feeling strong enough?

- Explore your reasons for wanting to lose weight. These are what will keep you going even when you don't feel like it.
- Assess your eating habits and establish your reasons for overeating or indulging in the wrong foods.
- It is assumed that you have the desire to get healthier and lose weight. Here, you state clearly and positively to yourself what you want, and then decide that you will accomplish it with

persistence. Use the self-hypnosis routine explained above to drive this point into your subconscious mind.

- Determine your motivation for the desired results, and how you will know when you've accomplished the goal. How will you feel, what you will see, and what are you likely to hear when you achieve your goal.

- Devote the first session of self-hypnosis to making the ultimate decision about your weight. Note that you must never have any doubt in your mind about your challenge to lose weight.

- Plan your meals every day. Weigh yourself frequently to monitor your progress as well. However, do not be paranoid about weighing yourself as this can actually negatively affect your progress.

- Repeat to yourself every day that you are getting to your ideal weight, that you've developed new, sensible eating habits, and that you are no longer prone to temptation.

- Think positively and provide positive affirmations in your self-induced hypnotic state.

Tweak Your Lifestyle

Every little thing counts. This is an important thing to note if you want to lose weight and slim down. Making a few changes in your regular daily activities can help you burn more calories.

- Walk more
- Use the stairs instead of the escalator or elevator if you're just going up or down a floor or two.

- Park your car a mile away from your destination and walk the rest of the way. You can also walk briskly to burn more calories.
- During your rest day, make it more active by taking your dog for a long walk in the park.
- If you need to travel a few blocks, save gas and avoid traffic by walking. For greater distances, dust off that old bike and pedal your way to your destination.
- Watch how and what you eat
- A big breakfast kicks your body into hyper metabolism mode so you should not skip the first meal of the day.
- Brushing after a meal signals your brain that you've finished eating, making you crave less until your next scheduled meal.
- If you need to get food from a restaurant, make your order to-go so you won't get tempted by their other offerings.
- Plan your meals for the week, so you can count how many calories you are consuming in a day.
- Make quick, healthy meals so you save time. There are thousands of recipes out there. Do some research?
- Eat at a table, not in your car. Drive-thru food is almost always greasy and full of unhealthy carbohydrates.
- Put more leaves, like arugula and alfalfa sprouts on your meals to give you more fiber and make you eat less.
- Order the smallest meal size if you really need to eat fast food.
- Start your meal with a vegetable salad. Dip the salad into the dressing instead of pouring it on.

- For a midnight snack, munch on protein bars or just drink a glass of skim milk.
- Eat before you go to the grocery to keep yourself from being tempted by food items that you don't really plan to buy.
- Clean out your pantry by taking out food items that won't help you with your fitness goals.

The whole idea in the tweaks mentioned is that you should eat less and move more. You may be able to think of additional tweaks.

Chapter 28
Strategies and Mind Exercises

When we think of weight management, our minds often go to diet and exercise. What's more important than hitting the gym is exercising our brain? If we make sure that the most important organ in our body is taken care of, we can be certain that other healthy habits will soon follow. You can diet, exercise, and do everything else you need to lose weight, but if you continually distract, deflect, or flat out avoid your problems and root issues, you will never find true happiness. The happier you are and the more aware you can be of your mental health, the better it will be in the end which will also lead to an overall better quality of life.

Keep a Journal

Keeping a journey is a healthy habit for many people no matter what their goals, but it's important for someone that wants to lose weight as well. By writing down your different portion measurements and exercise habits, you can better ensure that you'll have a basis for evaluation. When this is done, you can predict future problems that might keep you from your goals by looking back on the days of recorded mistakes or slipups. You can see what kinds of schedules and structures aren't working so you can create better habits in the end. The more extensive your journaling, the better you'll be able to create your own research study of your weight-loss journey, meaning you can share your progress or use it as a structure for future diets.

Avoid the Scale

The biggest issue with weight-loss strugglers comes when they see the number on the scale. Someone that wants to lose ten pounds might get discouraged if they find they only lost nine. Sometimes, people might even have to gain weight before they end up losing a pound. By avoiding the scale altogether, certain failures and disappointments can be avoided as well.

Find a different way to track your progress. You can have monthly weigh-ins, but it shouldn't be something that should be checked once a day. Our weight fluctuates so much throughout our journey that it isn't worth stressing over on a daily basis. Any checking that happens more than once a day is also likely a bad habit; you're using it to distract yourself from a bigger issue.

The Calorie Myth

When many people diet, they focus too much on calories. They'll see that a certain snack pack only has a hundred calories, which means that it's good for you, right? Wrong. When we focus too much on how many calories are in something, we're failing to look at all the other factors that make up that product. Something with zero calories might include harmful chemicals or hidden substances that are bad for us. Something with a ton of calories might be avoided even though it has a large number of vitamins and necessary fiber.

Calories should still be considered, as the more calories you take in, the more you have to burn through exercise. They still shouldn't be a basis for what foods you decide to eat. If you focus too much on calories, you'll end up losing sight of other important issues. Remember that weight loss isn't about numbers. What's on the scale or on the nutrition package is important in making certain measurements, but they shouldn't be the definitive goals that you're creating on your weight-loss journey.

Talk About It

Keeping things in is never good. In fact, it can feel pretty awful. Those that are overweight might find themselves feeling embarrassed about their weight. Maybe they end up making excuses for themselves when they eat certain foods, verbalizing these reasons to others around them as a form of validation. "Oh, I'll just start my diet tomorrow," you might hear someone say as they sneak a few extra cupcakes from the dessert table. This kind of discussion can be counterintuitive. Instead, try talking about the issues and struggles you have rather than about the way you're going to make up for your problems later. You might find that you end up getting some great advice from a person that's going through a similar struggle.

It's important to be a good listener as well. Sometimes, people aren't looking for answers or advice when they're complaining about their issues. It's nice just to have someone to vent to every once in a while. By creating a discussion, you can more easily tackle the issues that are causing problems in your weight-loss journey.

Avoid telling people about your goal before you get on track, however. Talking about your feelings, emotions, and struggles is always a good thing. Sometimes it just takes saying a thing out loud for it to feel real. However, many people set themselves up for failure by sharing their goals too early. Those that post on social media about how they're going to lose weight are actually less likely to follow through with their goals. Stay silent with the majority in the beginning of your journey, confiding in just those you know you can rely on and trust.

Affirmations

Practicing affirmations is an important mindset strategy in weight loss. An affirmation is a type of positive reinforcement that helps in combating negative thoughts. Instead of telling yourself you're "no good" because you didn't follow through with a small goal, you should give yourself an affirmation such as "I am capable of continuing" to remind yourself of how powerful you really are. Below is a list of positive affirmations you should use in order to combat negative thoughts and improve overall encouragement:

1. I can do this. I am capable of losing weight and I have the ability to reach my goals.
2. I am exercising every day and eating healthy as often as possible. I am actually doing what I should be doing in order to achieve my goals.
3. If I can start my journey, I can finish it.

4. I do not need processed foods to feel happy. I can feel the same joy from cooking a healthy meal.
5. I have exercised before and can do it again. It is hard to start, but I know that once I do, I have what it takes to finish my exercise routine.
6. I am healing myself. I have been through challenging times and deserve to feel happy.
7. I am loved and am full of love.
8. I am losing weight to be healthy.
9. I am beautiful no matter what size. Skipping one day at the gym does not mean that I am not beautiful.
10. I am eating healthy food full of nourishment. I can feel the positive change in my body, and I know that I only have more to look forward to.

Time Management

The most important part of a weight-loss journey is time management. This doesn't mean setting a quick goal and achieving it as fast as possible. It's all about using time properly and understanding how long it takes actually to do something. We set ridiculous goals for ourselves in the hopes that we'll achieve something great, but what ends up happening is, as the end-date approaches, we become overwhelmed and are set up for disappointment. We have to be realistic with our time goals and consider all factors when making different plans.

Practice Patience

Patience is hard to achieve. Anyone that wants to lose weight hopes that they can just jump on the scale after eating a salad and see the number drop by double digits. We have to accept before starting a weight-loss journey that this will never happen. We won't be able just to lose the weight overnight.

Sometimes, patience is hard to have when exercising. Many people find themselves getting bored on treadmills or other machines that require repetitive activity for minutes at a time. Use different exercise methods that you find fun or entertaining, such as a dance class or going on an interesting trail run. If the gym is your only option, use the boring moments on machines as a way to meditate. Clear your head, not thinking of how much weight you want to lose or what else you have to do to get there. Just practice counting or focusing on a quiet place you find peace in, such as a beach or a park. Visualize this in order to find a place of meditation. It'll take practice, but you'll soon find that you can zone out and work hard if you just focus.

There is No Rush

Weight loss takes time; we can't emphasize that enough. Some diets and exercises will help you lose weight quicker than others, but overall, you're going to have to put in a lot of time to lose weight. Remember not to feel too rushed throughout this journey. You have to be strict and consistent actually to see results, but there's no point in forcing yourself into ridiculous time constraints. If you cause yourself anxiety over certain dates, you might feel the need to stress-eat or go through dangerous dieting practices to get there.

Set Small Goals

Instead of looking at a wedding coming up in a couple of months as your goal for losing weight, instead, use that as a small milestone. Many of us get worried looking at the future, thinking of things coming up as the time limits for which we have to lose weight. Maybe it's March and you only have a couple months until swimsuit season. Instead of going on a diet to lose thirty pounds in three months, use the beginning of summer as a small milestone in your journey. Aim, instead, to be healthier and more confident by the time summer comes, rather than giving yourself a ridiculous goal that you don't even know if you can achieve.

Don't Wait for Monday

Many people have an unhealthy perceptive of dieting when looking at certain periods of time. Maybe it's a Tuesday, and so they tell themselves that next Monday is going to be the date to start dieting. In preparation for that date, that same person might make sure to eat all the junk in their house to make sure temptation is removed. But then, by the time Monday comes, something else happens that delays it further.

Even worse, maybe it's Sunday night and you decide that since tomorrow is Monday, you're going to start your diet right now. But then, Tuesday comes, and the diet doesn't start, so you feel discouraged and you count that as just another time that you failed! Don't do this! Instead, set a starting point much further into the future. Find a date two weeks away, whether it's on a Monday, the first of the month, or just a random Wednesday. That way, you can prepare for the official diet-start date. This way, you can practice as the actual date approaches.

Conclusion

Let's look back at our progress and then paying it forward to others. Ensure you revisit all the things you subscribed to while reading this book. Continue eating better all day. You'll feel better, look better, achieve your goals, and have a better quality of life. Assuming you've read and understood all the content in this book, chances are that you've realized your habits and applying core solutions to overcoming obstacles while holding yourself accountable, you have Paid attention to yourself, your purpose, unique talents, and dreams. By automating your food and water, cutting out unhealthy sugar, alcohol and white carbs, adding protein, Greek yogurt or other probiotics, produce and healthy fats.

Choose to continue with the same eating habit all your life. Focus on a healthy weight; stay with silence. Visualize your step and take steps that are going to get you to where you want to be. Destabilize procrastination, stress, comfort zone- you will go farther at a fast pace. Organize your kitchen and automate your food. Be a reader; Read positive affirmations aloud every day. Pursue your goals, including your fitness and health goals that will utilize your talents and passions and keep you on the healthy fit journey. Rest on weekends and refollow the process.

Focus on your activities, journalize your progress, thoughts, and move on. Record your success, nature; they will guide you in thinking and solving stress, among other problems. You will not only make an impact on yourself but also on the people around you. Make use of productivity apps on the internet to guide you through.

While writing your journal, consider how you've grown physically, mentally, spiritually, and emotionally or socially. Think about how one area has positively affected other areas. If some things haven't worked out for you, spend some time forgiving other people, forgiving yourself so you can move on. Giving makes living worthwhile.

Albert Einstein believed that a life shared with others is worthy. We have people out there who need you, remember not to hoard your successes. Share your success. Share your new-found recipes, your attitude, and your habits. Share what you have learned with others. In all your undertakings, know that you can't change other people but yourself, therefore, be mindful. Reflect on your changes and Put yourself on the back today and every day. Be grateful and live your life as a champion.

Make it a reality on your mind the fact that the journey to a healthy life and weight loss is long and has many challenges. Pieces of Stuff we consider more important in life require our full cooperation towards them. Just because you are facing problems in your Wight loss journey, it does not mean that you should stop, instead show and prove the whole world how good your ability to handle constant challenges is — training your brain to know that eating healthy food together with functional exercises can work miracles. Make it your choice and not something you are forced to do by a third party. Always tell yourself that weight loss is a long process and not an event. Take every day of your days to celebrate your achievements because these achievements are what piles up to massive victory. Make a list of stuff you would like to change when you get healthy they may be Small size-clothes, being able to accumulate enough energy, participating in your most loved sports you have been admiring for a more extended period, feeling self-assured. Make these tips your number one source of empowerment; you will end up completing your 30 days even without noticing.

You have made it, or you are about to make it. The journey has been unbelievable. And by now, you must be having a story to tell. Concentrate on finishing strongly. Keep up the excellent eating design you have adopted. Remember, you are not working on temporary changes but long term goals. Therefore, lifestyle changes should not be stopped when the weight is lost. Remind yourself always of essential habits that are easier to follow daily. They include; trusting yourself and the process by acknowledging that the real change lies in your hands. Stop complacency, arise, and walk around for at least thirty minutes away. Your breakfast is the most important meal you deserve. Eat your breakfast like a queen. For each diet, you take, add a few proteins and natural fats. Let hunger not kill you, eat more, but just what is recommended, bring snacks and other meals 3- five times a day. Have more veggies and fruits like 5-6 rounds in 24 hours. Almost 90% of Americans do not receive enough vegetables and fruits to their satisfaction. Remember, Apple will not make you grow fat. Substitute salt. You will be shocked by the sweet taste of food once you stop consuming salt. Regain your original feeling you will differentiate natural flavorings from artificial flavors. Just brainstorm how those older adults managed to eat their food without salt or modern-day characters. Characters are not suitable for your health. Drink a lot of water in a day. Let water be your number one drink. Avoid soft drinks and other energy drinks, and they are slowly killing you. Drink a lot of water in the morning after getting out of your bed. Your body will be fresh from morning to evening. Have a journal, and be realistic with it. Take charge of what you write and be responsible.

We all have common questions concerning diets. They touch everybody from doctors to nurses. Must you always have to be on a diet? Well, your body deserves healthy food with feeling good and looking well, and by automating the process, it should make it a no brainer. What if you don't grow as successful as you hoped? Failure is part of life. Accept and move on. Repeat the process. Consider what worked for you and make some changes to what didn't work. Like Emerson, when you persist in doing something, it becomes easier. Be on the move, explore, learn, and grow. Make plans and commit to them.

Eat protein, Greek yogurt, and they will prevent disease and make you healthy. Adopt healthy fats and carbs, change to local produce, Greek yogurt. Lastly, take what you have gained from this book, combining it with your skills, ability, and purpose; you will make significant steps and move forward.

What if I adopt herbs and other commercial products to lose weight? Well, you are a grown-up, and you know how pharmaceuticals maximize more profits from our health. They sell what will harm us more so that we back for more of their products, thereby making more profits at the expense of our health. Those pills are temporary pleasure generators. There is no magic in that stuff. There is nothing like fat absorbers. You hold the key to fat absorption. When they are useful, you can tell that they are, and when they are safe, they do not offer the required solution. To tackle your overweight, you have to deal with the problem directly. Make changes in your life. These are some remedies;

Acai berries: being that all seeds are antioxidants, acai berries from Brazil has zero or no weight loss benefit on the human body. No research has been carried to proving how such berries benefits in weight loss, clean intestines, improve sexual life, acne, or popular lies accompanying their advertisement. They are very expensive and exist in tablet forms, juice forms, and other forms. They beat logic and is only fair for profit.

Garcinia cambogia; many theories have been developed and more studies done by researchers to test the performance of Garcinia. The results have been unimpressive. According to a survey conducted on one hundred and thirty-five participants. They were given 1500 milligrams of Garcinia cambogia daily or placebo. They were then put in a diet with a small calorie content and fiber-rich intake. After three months, participants under placebo recorded a decline in weight. For Garcinia cambogia participants, no weight loss was recorded. From the study, it is evident that Garcinia cambogia has no business in weight loss.

Chitosan: they are derivative of crustacean's covers. Business-people advertise as a fat absorber when it is believed to suck fats in the intestine. Existing research shows that one needs to consume a lot of Chitosan daily to record a cut in fat absorption rate. The amount of fat absorbed is minimal in quantity. Chitosan does not promote weight cut.

The dra alkaloids: it is natural .it is at the same time a stimulant with minimal effect on appetite. FDA has advised against consuming products containing lots of Ephedra alkaloids. The user of these products is at high risk of getting diseases like stomach-ache, heart diseases, mental problems, liver malfunction, and depression. Even when consumed in low quantity, Ephedra has broad adverse effects on the body, and it would be good if you avoid it. It does not play any role in losing weight.

What is the notion of drugs helping in losing weight? Remember, for you to lose and maintain your weight, you must have long term goals and employ positive life change in all your life. Even if those drugs produce god results, you will be advised to use them all your life. Who loves taking drugs till their death day! When you stop taking them, the results start to be harmful, and your life will deteriorate, and you will gain more weight. Losing weight revolves around your diet. Your diet determines your health. Some drugs acting as appetite suppressants have been popular in the recent past. Their dangers have also spread. They cannot be adopted for long term effects; therefore, it would be unfair to advise you on taking these drugs.

According to Joel Fuhrman, FDA has approved two drugs for weight loss and includes; "Meridia and Xenical. Meridia can cause pains, sleeplessness, constipation, thirsty mouth, and high blood pressure. Their positive effects are minimal. Xenical, the fat preventer, causes lower stomach pains and watery feces. It decreases the immersion of fats in vitamins. Such vitamins are; vitamin C, vitamin E, and vitamin K."

Will I eat junk food again? You can consume what you feel like eating at some moments, but make sure you do not let such attitude mature. Be very strict the first two weeks to record the weight you are to lose by following your plan. The temptation is real. You will be tempted to eat junk food regularly. Resist such temptation and keep those foods away from your kitchen. Just taste them once if it is a must but outside your apartment. Again, relate with a friend who will be supportive in your journey to a healthy life.

GASTRIC BAND HYPNOSIS FOR WEIGHT LOSS:

Sharpen your mind to shape your body. rapid weight loss self-hypnosis to Stop Food Addiction, burn fat quickly and Eat Healthy, with Permanent Results.

Introduction

The gastric band (also known as a lap band) has become an increasingly common surgical procedure for those who want to lose weight. A band is fitted around the stomach and inflated to greatly minimize stomach capacity. This means the patient eats less food, resulting in fast and permanent weight loss.

However, gastric band surgery is not risk-free. In any surgery something goes wrong, there is always the inherent danger, but there are also certain problems that the lap band can directly cause.

This involves a slipped band (which may result in excessive or inadequate stomach capacity), acid reflux, nausea, vomiting, diarrhea, regurgitation, blockages, and other problems. And while the findings are good, there are certainly secret risks. Yet wouldn't it be nice to duplicate the gastric band's performance without any of the risks?

Okay, there's definitely a way. Recently, hypnotherapists successfully repeated the lap band treatment with hypnotic suggestions. No scalpels, anesthetics, scars— just pure mind control. Because of its safe and efficient existence, gastric band hypnotherapy has become the new weight-loss craze.

A quick Google search shows hundreds of happy patients who have undergone hypnotherapy and lost much of their excess weight.

Why does it work, though?

To understand how gastric band hypnotherapy functions, we must first look at hypnosis and mental influence.

Although human mind awareness is far from complete, the most welcoming theory is that the mind consists of two major components— the conscious and the subconscious. You'll be most familiar with the idea of conscious mind, because that's where your daily style of thinking comes from.

Whenever you think "I'm thirsty, I should go get a drink" or something similar that's your conscious mind at work.

Your subconscious mind is far deeper and stronger. It governs all those instinctive behaviors and responses you don't even think about, your routines, impulses and phobias. Hypnosis operates on the subconscious mind. Hypnosis primes the subconscious, able to consider suggestions.

Now we understand how hypnosis works, it is a little clearer how hypnotherapy works. A hypnotherapist creates a hypnotic state in their client and then speaks to them as if it really occurs via the gastric band procedure.

There is no actual physical discomfort or anything, but the subconscious mind finds differentiating between fantasy and reality very difficult. That's why sometimes very strong dreams seem too real.

When the subconscious mind thinks the body has a gastric band fitted, it will behave as though you have one fitted. This means you'll feel satisfied faster, eat slower, and consume fewer meals. This naturally leads to very successful weight loss.

Besides being safer than surgery, gastric band hypnotherapy is often much more convenient-approximately ten times less costly than surgery.

Many audio packs provided by professional hypnotherapists have the very same session on CD or MP3 and are much less costly as the hypnotherapist only has to record the session once with certain clients. And if you're talking about gastric band surgery, the natural form of hypnotherapy may well be worth your consideration.

Hypnotic Gastric Banding Therapy

The therapist opens the subconscious mind to feedback and attempts not to change an old pattern, but to create a new one.

The hypnotherapist will indicate to your subconscious mind that you simply have a stomach-fitted surgical band and that your stomach is just the size of a golf ball. The hypnotherapist should speak to you about the process.

Your experience will begin with the therapist bringing you through a very calm state of mind, and you are led through all the sounds of the hospital that one would expect to hear, such as the voices and noises wheeling down the hospital's corridors on the way to the operating theatre.

You must move through in-hospital doctors and nurses, bangs and clangs of sterile stainless-steel bowls and instruments, and a bustling metropolitan hospital's general everyday noise.

The gurney (operating trolley) then stops when you enter the operating room, and the nurse asks if you are ready for surgery. You respond "Yes," so the anesthetist moves forward to administer anesthetic.

You can hear people talking about the operation of the gastric band, you can hear alarms beeping, and you feel surgically operated on. The hypnotic banding weight loss treatment takes you through the whole surgical cycle. Y

you are then brought back into the recovery room after the procedure, when the doctor takes you back into the moment, at this stage many people actually check their stomach to check whether they have had procedure, because their mind strongly assumes they already have a gastric band fitted and they still feel their stomach is limited to eating smaller quantities.

Gastric band surgery, as you probably already know, is a common weight loss choice. Many very overweight and obese individuals underwent surgery and lost hundreds of pounds and kilos successfully. Hypnosis-assisted weight loss is another choice for Gastric Lap Band Surgery.

Patients who have undergone the hypnotic version feel that they've actually had the surgery, as I mentioned many of them even raise their shirts to see if they've had an incision after the surgery they think they've just had, the hypnotherapist's thought deep inside their subconscious is so strong that people find it hard to believe they haven't.

Hypnotic gastric banding or weight loss with hypnosis support is pain-free and also a healthy way to have gastric band surgery. There is an alternative to spending significant sums of money on surgery, and the sometimes-prolonged recovery period is not required. You have all the surgery advantages, but without the complications.

As many TV shows feature them, Hypnotic Gastric Banding is increasingly common. Hypnosis weight loss is a fantastic option and many clients will testify to having lost hundreds of pounds from this type of therapy.

Enjoy opening your mind and discovering life's various possibilities. Hypnotherapy is now commonly recognized and is growing as the impressive outcomes become more well-known and more physicians, many in the medical community and natural therapists see and support the therapies available using hypnotherapy.

Chapter 1:
Self – Hypnosis

Next, we will look at the art of manipulating your conscious and rewiring your suobconscious to lose weight with the following six steps.

Step 1: Study or adjust your schedule to find time when you won't be distracted by your surroundings. This is a time set out for yourself where you are required to focus for 30 to 60 minutes to allow yourself to enter a trance state of mind where you feel completely relaxed and content without any interruptions.

Step 2: Set a weight loss intention to reach your goals, but rather than only focusing on how much weight you want to lose, focus on all the benefits that you will reap because of it. Since a weight loss journey is also considered to be a positive and reconstructive journey, make certain you allow space for focusing on the value you place on your body. Placing value on our bodies is extremely important and helpful. It can teach us respect and motivate a greater reason behind perseverance to complete what we set out to do. Visualizing how much weight you'd like to lose in a reasonable period will set the tone for your goal before you begin. Make sure you say your goal out loud to ensure that your intention is set.

Step 3: Visualize your end-goal. What does your body look like and what size are you? How do you feel once you get closer to your goal? Also focus on how you feel once you've reached your goal. Do you feel fulfilled and accomplished? Focus on the benefits you will reap once you've reached your goal, as well as the possibilities that will follow.

Step 4: Look the part. Close your eyes and enter a state of relaxation. Much like with meditation, your mind must be quiet and calm. Now you can engage in deep breathing for up to three minutes and choose your breathing technique, either the diaphragmatic technique or the Buteyko breathing technique. Make sure you continue to breathe until you feel calm and relaxed throughout your entire body. Now relax your body, you've entered a trance state of mind.

Step 5: Visualize yourself reaching your goal in a trance state of mind. How good do you feel in your skin now that you've reached your goal weight? Do you miss your bad habits, and do you feel better now that you've left them behind? Do people look up to you for losing weight? Focus on the positivity surrounding the fact that you've accomplished something you possibly didn't think was possible before. Continuing with this state of mind will allow you to change your behavior and increase the desire for you to implement change into your life.

Step 6: Return to your present state with ease, and don't rush it. You are in a relaxed state of mind and you should focus on bringing the feelings back to your reality. By doing this session daily and reminding yourself of how you feel, you will be able to adjust your mindset and increase the possibility of losing weight. You will receive new energy for taking on obstacles in your life and be able to make behavioral modifications where it is necessary.

Why weight loss hypnotherapy is for you?

Have you ever thought about food as your friend?

Have you ever thought about your friends and family as a priority?

If you answer both of these questions honestly, you'll come to find that food is supposed to be your friend. Thinking of it in that way, you will surely treat it with more respect. Given that we only get one body and that our bill of health deteriorates over time, we are most definitely obliged to look after ourselves. The same goes for kicking bad habits like smoking, consuming too much alcohol, possibly consuming mind-altering drugs, and even other negative factors like depriving yourself of sleep.

Hypnosis is all about bettering yourself, and if you can reach a state where you are focused on improving your health and feel willing to do so daily, you will finally change your mindset toward food, exercise, and bad habits.

Eating food that is beneficial for your health will become second nature.

Setting an attainable goal for yourself, like reaching 21-days of eating clean, will eventually lead to everything that follows thereafter if you manage to stick to self-hypnosis. Twenty-one days of consistency will allow you to create new habits and familiarities, which will keep you on track even after you've reached your weight loss goals. After a while, eating healthily won't feel like a punishment, but rather like a reward.

You will feel better by eating better, but also eating less

If you're like most people, you probably love eating and food in general, right? Just because you follow a diet and workout routine, does not mean that you can't enjoy your food. However, keeping in mind that you have three meals a day, and possibly one or two snacks, you should be mindful that your body doesn't need too much food. If our stomach is the size of your two hands clasped together in a fist, then where does the rest of the food you consume go? It gets deposited as fat storage in your body, which is exactly what you don't want. Focus on mindful eating and listen to your body. You will also find that eating less actually satisfy you more.

It shifts your attitude tremendously

One of the biggest changes hypnosis implements is your mindset toward eating and exercising. While many individuals who engage in hypnosis do it to control their eating habits, there's a lot of change to be made to most people's sedentary lifestyles.

You are a human and you are designed to move, to hunt, to gather.

If you sit down all day and don't push your body out of its comfort zone, it will waste away and die.

Chapter 2:
What is Hypnosis?

Both hypnosis and meditation do offer a deeply relaxing, calming, and an extremely beneficial state of mind, which plays a significant role in helping you to get through your day. Besides, hypnosis and meditation are the keys to unusual calmness and positivity as you start to address psychological, physical, and social issues.

The distinction between meditation and hypnosis is distorted because they are wrapped around the same state of mind, but they have different belief systems in their purest form. Hypnosis is a common natural state of mind whereby you tend to concentrate on a single thought, while meditation is a means that you use to enter into a hypnotic state.

Meditation is often characterized by relaxation and visualization, especially when you are trying to find tranquility, and reconnect with your personality, or seek guidance on an issue. Notably, this form of meditation has a pure purpose, structure, and it makes use of visualization, to help shape your life, which is referred to as self-hypnosis.

Combinations of the two states of relaxation both provide incredible results as they help to take control of your mind and perception. Meditation is effective as it helps to empty the mind and free it of all thoughts, while hypnosis goal in mind is to either help to overcome an obstacle, develop confidence, or help you to rediscover your potential. It does not matter if you practice meditation or hypnosis, so long as it is pleasant and it offers a positive experience, then it's great.

These two states of mind are very vital to you if you wish to lead a fulfilled and happier life.

How They Work

Normally, your conscious mind usually makes you aware of your thought processes. So, you only tend to think about the situations that you are facing and make the right choice of words and actions to overcome those situations. Also, the subconscious mind is a huge aspect of your thoughts as it functions "behind the scenes" and works closely with the conscious mind.

For instance, if you're consciously trying to remember where you placed your keys, the subconscious mind accesses the information reservoir in your subconscious mind to help you to find exactly where you placed your keys. Also, the subconscious mind helps you to complete tasks that seem automatic, like breathing and constructing sentences.

 Hypnosis and meditation are the most natural ways for you to be able to directly access your subconscious mind, enhance your thought process, and act as the brain behind every operation. The conscious mind is most active when you are awake because it helps to evaluate your thoughts and determines which ideas to put into action. They are responsible for processing the acquired information that the subconscious mind needs. On the contrary, the subconscious mind is the one in control whenever you fall asleep. At that moment, it renders the conscious mind ineffective for your thinking.

Hypnosis and meditation are characterized by deep and focused exercises and relaxation, which subdues and calm the conscious mind to a much less active role as in the sleep state although you are still aware of the happenings in your environment, as they both deactivate the conscious mind and work directly with the subconscious mind.

This subconscious state of mind allows you to be able to control the brain and gain access to your information reservoir, where you could change your perception about an impending task. Also, it allows you to become more creative as it induces your impulses and imagination. Hypnosis and meditation work together through many different mechanisms. These techniques include emotion, change in self-perspective, body awareness, and attention regulation.

These components are necessary for helping with all the various aspects of your life, and when combined together, the cumulative process thus leads to an enhanced self-regulation capacity. If you lack this capacity on a personal level, then it will cause psychological suffering and distress for you. So, practicing meditation plays a significant role in helping you to develop command over the mind, and makes you capable of controlling your thoughts, when you're done meditating.

The main aim of practicing hypnosis and meditation is to help control your thoughts and achieve the things that seem impossible to achieve through the conscious mind.

The Best Time for Hypnosis and Meditation

To succeed in these practices, you should create a routine that will help to keep you on track as you practice often. These practices are very similar to the things that require daily commitment as one of the obvious parts of achieving your results.

The more you hypnotize and meditate, the more you will be able to take charge of your body. Daily practices are recommended so that you will be able to choose the best time for you, depending on your work schedule and lifestyle. It's better to practice meditation and hypnosis when waking up, during the lunchtime break, or before you sleep.

Also, the practice is suitable to do during morning break or immediately after you finish working. No matter your preferences, you should ensure that the time you choose fits into your lifestyle.

You do not have to use too much time to meditate because if you do, then you are going to lose interest or fall asleep. Also, it's advisable to practice sessions of meditation for around 15-20 minutes, two to three times daily in a quiet and comfortable place. Initially, you will not notice any significant results, but you have to realize that everything in life gets better with practice.

There are different ways of learning meditation, but the most important thing in meditation is the ability to be able to imagine and think about the changes that you are expecting to get in your life. Therefore, it does not matter whether you can visualize it or not; you have to make it a routine so that you will be able to transform your conscious mind and address any complex issue.

Hypnosis and meditation greatly help to enhance your feelings and make it easy for you to deal with all psychological problems like anxiety, stress, and depression. Also, if you want to experience a drastic weight loss and be able to control your eating habits, then you should incorporate hypnosis and meditation into your plan and make it a regular practice. You can practice meditation at anytime and anywhere, as long as you stay inactive, and you don't experience any interruptions.

The Practical Guide to using hypnosis for weight loss

It is worth knowing that your unconscious thoughts are purely shaped by your experiences, memories, and expectations. These aspects help to drive your conscious actions without you even realizing it. Your subconscious mind normally sets you up to fail; that's why it's difficult for you to be able to address your bad habits.

Hypnosis is critical in helping to update and alter those negative thoughts, thus making it possible for you to be able to critical conditions like chronic pain, substance abuse, and weight loss. When you begin to train your mind to think differently about setting goals and challenges, then you will be able to get rid of those thoughts that are making you to self-sabotage. Your mind will become suggestible when you're in a trance state, which will then enable you to be able to access and influence your powerful subconscious assumptions. So, by following this guide, you will be able to take positive actions towards the changes that you have successfully set for yourself.

Hypnosis session for weight loss

So now you can relax and take this time to wind yourself down and allow all those tensions to start flowing out and disappearing. So just bring to mind to remember that hypnosis is just self-hypnosis, as you're reading now, that this is not something that someone will be able to do for you. Because hypnosis is simply a state of deep relaxation, which successfully helps you to bypasses your own critical factors so that the suggestions that are beneficial to your true self will be readily received and accepted by your deeper unconscious mind.

After all, trance is an everyday natural calming experience, and you're entering into that experience easily and effortlessly.

The most important thing to realize is that you should bring to your mind, relaxation, and protective magical thinking practices each day in your waking state because you know that the practice imprints it in your mind. And as time goes by, it becomes easier for you to be able to gain the benefits of these experiences, which helps to promote self-acceptance.

Once they become permanently fixed into your mind, you will experience some positive changes in your life, and they will become active by helping you to create positive changes in your life that are for your benefit, and they will lead you forward towards a real realization of those changes. And as you speak directly to the deeper inner part of the self that controls your eating habits and weight, you will realize that you have been eating more food than the food that your body wants or needs. And also, you will realize that your mind controls your eating habits.

Now just seeing all those levers that you can adjust, you can then choose which one to use because you know that you have the power over your weight and your eating habits. And also, you know what you're eating. The exact time and amount that you choose to eat are totally controlled in this place, which is the deeper part of your authentic self.

This part of the body is not your stomach or your appetite, but it really controls your food, but it is your own mind, and you get to ask that aspect of yourself beginning today, to develop new habits for yourself. And set new positive goals for yourself because you are laying a mental foundation for yourself, who is now a cheerful, attractive, positive, and authentic you. The great importance to this new you and to your healthy, active, and attractive body is that you are eating less food, and you're happier.

The more you smile, and the more relaxed you are, the better you will look and the better you will feel. Also, you will be able to find satisfaction in eating less and pride yourself in knowing that each time you do so, you are rewarding your slimmer, healthier, and natural self. And you will know that the slimmer you are deep within you as you exercise, this new strength will grow. And as you eat healthily and sensibly, you will find yourself filling satisfied, and you will discover that the exercise makes it more reinforce and more natural towards your authentic identity.

Because it is like using and strengthening your muscles to become stronger and stronger, now eating sensibly becomes easier, easier, in a practical, and the positive way means that you are mentally asking your body the foods it needs, and then you are taking the time to listen to your own body quietly.

238

Chapter 3:

Positive Self Talk vs. Negative Self Talk

To reach your potential, you have to let go of some habits and some of the people you hang with. The most interesting thing about this is that many people have greatness locked up inside of them, all that they needed is to encounter someone that will unleash the beast and set them on the path of success. Many never met such people; many gave up too soon; many were even discouraged by friends. But the only way to unlocking your full potential is by discovering that you have such potential in the first place. It is after you have made this discovery that you can then move on to the next stage of development, which is to look out for ways that you can get leverage this greatness in you with life opportunities.

The main idea behind this kind of reasoning is that you have to look inward and look for ways to develop yourself. Nobody will help you if you refuse to help yourself. The earlier you realize this, the better it is. They significantly influence the level of accomplishment at each progression:

- Positive Thinking and Behavior
- Visualization
- Positive Self-Talk
- Affirmation Statements
- Dynamic Goal Setting
- Positive Action

- Assertive Behavior
- Success Strategies

These nine success strategies and behaviors are significant professional enhancers that help you to change objectives into real factors. Give close consideration to any that are new thoughts for you. They give wide-running advantages, and you can utilize them to:

☐   Create and support your internal drive

☐   Increase your certainty

☐   Provide mental and physical vitality

☐   Guide you toward objectives

Follow these means to frame the propensity for positive intuition and to help your prosperity. Intentionally spur yourself consistently. Consider yourself fruitful and expect positive results for all that you endeavor. By practicing these inspirational desire attitude until it turns into a propensity decision making process will be impacted to a great extent by this positive vitality. The propensity will assist you with arriving at your full potential.

Reflect on past victories helps, too, as this helps you to concentrate on past triumphs to help yourself to remember your capacities, and this boosts your ability to accomplish your objectives. For instance, nobody is ever brought into the world, realizing how to ride a bike or how to utilize a P.C. programming program. Through preparing, practice, and experimentation, you ace new capacities. During the experimentation periods of improvement, help yourself to remember past victories; see botches as a major aspect of the common expectation to absorb information. Proceed until you accomplish the outcome you need, and this reminds you that you have the necessary skillset to prevail since you have done it before and can also do it once more.

Certain affirmation statements are necessary for self-explanations or suggestions to help accomplish objectives. They are certain messages with a punch, "mental guard stickers," to persuade your psyche to work for you. The accompanying rules disclose how to utilize this amazing mental update strategy:

Offer the expression in the first person

Express yourself decidedly: The psyche acknowledges reality in the words you give it. Utilize positive words as it were.

Forget about negative words: For instance, this statement is negative: "I will be apprehensive during my meeting," while this other statement that's saying the same thing sounds positive: "I will be quiet and confident during my meeting.

Incorporate a positive feeling: An expression that triggers a positive feeling reinforces a sense of determination. As a model, you could say: "My objective is important, and it energizes me."

Stop Negative Self-Talk: You might rush to bother yourself since you need to be great. Be that as it may, negative self-talk is harming on the grounds that the inner mind truly accepts what you state about yourself. In case you get yourself utilizing negative self-talk, stop, and rethink. Take out the negative words. Concentrate rather on the best strategy you can take and do it.

Make positive correspondence a propensity: Concentrate on the positive in objective articulations, self-talk, and all interchanges. Think about the accompanying expressions and notice how the positive words pass on certainty, duty, and energy.

Set an objective and stick to it

Characterize your objectives unmistakably by having it recorded as a hard copy. Recording your objectives/goal improves the probability of accomplishing them by 80 percent! Composing objectives build your feeling of duty, explains required strides in the accomplishment procedure, and encourages you to recollect significant subtleties. Make the advantages (to you and others) of accomplishing objectives clear and distinct. This is a solid spark. It gives you a clear understanding of what you need to do to accomplish your aim. Furthermore, be sure to characterize the reason for your objectives. Connect your objectives to a functional, explicit reason. To support your own inspiration, base your objectives on motivation, not simply rationale. To make this easier, you can incorporate educators, books, preparing, individuals who urge you to drive forward, gifted mentors or coaches, and printed and online research materials. Finally, build up an activity plan, set cutoff times, and act. Build up sub-objectives. Partition every primary objective into consistent, dynamic advances—set cutoff times for finishing each progression and complete strides on schedule.

CHAPTER 4:
Subconscious Mind

What We Plant in Our Subconscious Mind

Grace's naturally magnificent charm and beauty brought her a complete scholarship to a prestigious modelling college. She fell out after six weeks because her weight ballooned to more than two hundred pounds, in which it stayed for another fifteen years regardless of persistent weight reduction attempts. Jack, fifty years older, was overweight since high school, even though playing sports, doing regular exercise, also creating many efforts at weight reduction. Whenever his weight starts to fall, he feels fearful until he regains the pounds.

Mary has won and gained the same twenty-five pounds throughout her adult life. She knows the routine and activates; however, she feels so helpless to alter them and shed the pounds once and for everyone. Alex is a successful executive at a competitive tech industry that always struggles with his burden.

He works hard, makes a higher income, and will multitask better than many, but cannot restrain the size of the waist. Ted has been CEO of a global source firm. His friends saw as he moved from being a photograph of wellness to some health hazard as a result of excessive weight reduction. Grace, Jack, Mary, Alex, along with Ted, are actual cases we found in treatment for weight loss with hypnosis.

Like many other people, these folks once believed that food and eating were the issues causing their surplus fat. We'll have a look at how inherent psychological problems are expressed in a way that triggers and keep excess fat. We'll learn more about using hypnosis to discover the use of feelings and burden. We're not likely to speak about eating disorders--like bulimia, anorexia, and pica--or even other hurtful behaviors.

The Mind-Body Mirror

Considering these are out of our mind-body medication practice, let's briefly look at a few of the standard methods that physical ailments are created by the mind-body. There are various examples where suppressed and repressed emotions locate saying by manifesting as physical symptoms and ailments.

Emotions and psychological conflicts that Aren't consciously acknowledged, voiced, or Provided voice mayor will be voiced from the body. Here's a pervasive case. When anger isn't recognized and expressed, it can lead to muscles in your head, neck, and shoulders to tighten up and stressed, which consequently makes a pressure headache. It is the literal manifestation of something or somebody that's a pain in the throat. Another individual experiencing the very same feelings of anger may be burning over the circumstance, also expertise nausea, nausea, or an illness.

Your skin is the organ that's quite responsive to feelings, and also a state of urticaria (hives) may erupt whenever somebody is getting under their skin or rubbing them the wrong manner or any time the individual is itching to say or do something, or even any emotion is erupting into the surface.

Your emotions are emotions, such as happy, sad, or mad. If feelings or emotions aren't expressed, the mind-body will reflect them in imaginative ways. Therapeutically, metaphors help us understand what the human body is expressing.

It can be a frequent encounter because most times, it isn't okay or advisable to admit and convey anger or other emotions. For instance, if your boss embarrasses you or gets an unreasonable request, then you can jeopardize your job if you voiced your anger. Instead,

You place it out of thoughts and go to another thing. Putting it from mind doesn't place it from human anatomy. Since you will notice from the cases of hypnosis used in treatment, feelings and psychological conflicts could be placed out of thoughts, but not always from the body. You're able to suppress feelings or repress them. Suppressing feelings is if you intentionally decide not to consider them. Repressing emotions occurs whenever your subconscious does this for you without having the advantage of choosing to perform it on yourself. We'd love to spell out the difference between thoughts and feelings. Ideas are thoughts, beliefs, ideas, and conclusions on your own conscious or "thinking thoughts." Feelings or emotions are expressed in your entire body.

They arise in a crude place deep within the brain known as the limbic system. Both ideas and feelings are "items" in the meaning they're not only in your thoughts. They involve power and chemistry, and they're transmitted and energetically throughout your nervous system along with other pathways inside the body. The chemical compounds called hormones, like dopamine, serotonin, noradrenaline, and acetylcholine, would be the common ones included.

If someone experiences mental sluggishness, then he can notice more psychological acuity if he comprises nuts, oatmeal, along with other choline-rich foods within his everyday decisions. Choline affirms the purposes of acetylcholine, which subsequently promotes memory and mental sharpness. For our purposes, we would like to highlight that these psychological and cognitive reactions and routines are real and happen to be analyzed.

Feelings or emotions comprise pain, anxiety, guilt, despair, joy, anger, pleasure, bliss, contentment, serene, stress, and isolation. Notice that "poor" and "good" aren't from the record of feelings. Though we may say "I feel awful" or "I'm great," these aren't emotions. These are conclusions about what you believe; however, they aren't feelings. More correctly, if you create these announcements you believe "I feel sick" or even "I feel well," that are approaches to explain how you're feeling, maybe not what you're feeling. Now, this is your only worth remembering: "Fat" isn't a feeling. Though folks say, "I feel fat," "fat" isn't a feeling.

Whenever someone says they're "feeling fat, then" it's a declaration about a feeling, like feeling fulfilled, filled, complete, or outside full. You could be thinking, "Why the big deal on the selection of words? I understand what I mean when I state that." The reason why we emphasize that is your feelings, as well as your voice about your emotions, are part of your own beliefs about yourself, and if you maintain these in understanding or talk them aloud, they're direct messages to your subconscious mind. Your mind-body finds all of it, and also long after it's from the mind (consciousness), it isn't from your own body's mind. You are going to want to select carefully what your goal will be to think and anticipate about your weight loss and exactly what and how you are feeling about it for it'll reflect it.

Saving Grace

One occurred to Grace that induced her to overlook her modelling college scholarship. She arrived at the office and expressed the desire to work with hypnosis to help her slim down. She clarified many different trials of weight loss methods which had been ineffective. Whenever she didn't lose fat, it'd return. She believed that there was "something" keeping her out of losing weight. In carrying her background, we discovered she had been thirty-six years older, married with three kids, ages eight, seven, seven and five. Her weight was always over two billion pounds for approximately fifteen decades.

She grew up at the mid-west at a fantastic family and also had three sisters. Grace explained himself as the only man in her household, having a weight issue. When asked regarding her weight record, she'd only say she "ate a lot." After finishing a thorough psychological and psychological evaluation, we proceeded to educate her about sculpting.

If she felt comfortable enough to move, we started with an induction method such as those on the sound with this publication. Grace relaxed readily into a trance country, wherein she had been absorbed in her thoughts and thoughts of a relaxing and enjoyable spectacle. As she pictured being on holiday with her loved ones, I provided hypnotic suggestions for her mind about letting her insight to the function or purpose of her extra body fat. In a couple of minutes, she seemed worried, and I asked her to explain what she was experiencing as she lasted.

She explained riding a train and also becoming the very first to arrive in the modelling school. The government office has been shut; however, a friendly janitor assisted her suitcases and unlocked the door to her delegated dining space. She was getting tearful and stressed as she continued talking. I assured her she would disrupt the squint in any moment or she would move more gradually and professionally, and that I informed her that she understood she had been at our office today as she recalled something which happened afterwards, fifteen decades back. Through her tears, she clarified the favorable janitor returning after that night, allowing himself to her chamber and hammering her.

The memory of the experience was rather exhausting and mentally draining for Grace. Discussing her following the trancework, I discovered it was nearly fifteen years since she'd thought about that adventure. She'd forgotten it. Initially, she opted to put this from her head, to curb this particular memory, but it had been put from her head so well that she'd forgotten that she forgot it. It had been repressed. She said this is the only real-time and location she had spoken to anybody about the encounter.

We spent a second session referring to her expertise in modelling faculty, and I requested her to earn some photos from this period. We used the photos to help her recall events so that she could chat about them at the security of treatment. She related that through the initial six months in school, her burden slowly improved, and she had been anxious, fearful, embarrassed, depressed, along with sleep-deprived. She didn't talk about the rape with anybody and moved home to wed her high school love.

He'd continuously accepted her for himself, and her burden was not a problem with him. Our counselling sessions demonstrated the goal of her excess body fat was a kind of defence. Her weight securely commanded her beauty so that she had been shielded from becoming the target of the following sexual assault. After she confessed, voiced, and revived the experience and feelings (fear, pity), Grace's weight loss plan was quite robust in cutting her dimension to wherever she felt joyful and secure. In her situation, we realize that the subconscious had been working out a role, and also there was a reason for the surplus weight.

It secured her and enabled her to feel secure. Though there was some time after she had been happy others found her appealing, the attack produced a panic that became linked to becoming captivating. After analyzing these feelings and eliminating this anxiety, she had been free to discharge her additional weight and feel secure when she felt appealing.

Chapter 5:
The Power of Visualization

Continual visualization directs your actions to reflect that of your mental image. This is why it is possible to acquire new skills with creative visualization. You can also use it to give yourself a new set of belief system. You only need to visualize yourself believing in the mental image you create without allowing any resistance into your visualization. You have to reprogram any negative and limiting beliefs if you are to achieve your goal. There are two main ways you can apply this kind of visualization in your life:

- Ensuring a healthy life and banishing bad habits
- Fostering strong relationships
- Manifesting financial abundance

Healthy Living and Banishing Bad Habits

Bad habits often start innocently; an over–indulgence during a holiday season that you do not seem to break even when the holidays are over, perfectly normal social situations that slowly get you hooked to the bad behavior, peer pressure, or unhealthy lifestyles. It may be drinking, smoking, over-eating, drug abuse or gambling. These are all bad habits that undermine any idea you have of making your body and mind healthy. However, to have and maintain a healthy mind you need to have a healthy and happy body.

a)   Use Creative Visualization to Heal

The best you can do for yourself is to use creative visualization. With the help of visualization, it is easy to break off any bad habits in your life and acquire the kind of perfect and healthy life you have been dreaming of. Creative visualization can help you quit smoking, reduce drinking and eating and return your body to better shape in no time.

Through creative visualization you an easily develop a positive attitude to improve your health. You only need to imagine yourself in that perfect body and health you dream of and you can easily make it into reality. According to researchers, they found out that an ill person is likely to change the situation by mentally picturing themselves combating their illness. Such action has been proven to reduce the severity of symptom in a patient and improve their quality and length of life.

However, always remember that when it comes to treating your illness with creative visualization you must use it with tested procedures and medicines. It is good to get the best professional care and advice to be able to take care of your medical problems fast and effectively. The power of creative thinking only hastens your recovery and enhances the effectiveness of conventional medicine and professional help. It increases your defense for battling any illness you may have.

The whole process of visualizing your well-being is a partnership between you, your doctor and your body. It is the doctor who determines what is ailing you and begins the medical treatment process to heal your condition. It is up to you to take the information you get from your doctor on where the problem is and pass it to your body. Through creative visualization you get your body to work on the problem as the same time you are receiving conventional medication. This is a process that can easily help you combat any serious and minor illness you have. It involves adopting a positive outlook on your health to keep your immune system in top shape.

b)   Use Creative Visualization to Build Strong Core Muscles

As you grow older your muscles weaken, especially if you are not active. A sedentary life makes your joints calcify and this often leads to osteoarthritis. When you are young and active you may not think about the aches and pain of joint problems. However, when you get to your middle ages these pains become more pronounced. What you need to do is to keep your muscles in good condition.

When using creative visualization, remember that it is impossible to build muscles simply by visualizing them. You need to get active if you want to develop your core muscles and be physically fit. Visualization helps to hasten the process and give you the motivation to keep your mind on the desired results and maintain it.

The benefits of toughening your core muscles can be realized through:

- Improved posture and less lower back pain
- Toned muscles that prevent the occurrence of back injuries
- Enhanced physical performance
- Less muscle aches
- Better balance made possible by having lengthened legs

According to physiotherapists and Pilates, the kind of physical and visualization exercise you engage in should emphasize to your body and unconscious mind the importance of keeping your muscles strong and fit to benefit you in all of the above-mentioned areas. They believe that this technique is the key to developing core stability. This is where your abdominal wall, lower back, diaphragm and pelvis are able to stabilize your body during movement.

How to Combine Physical Exercise with Creative Visualization

Step 1: Do abdominal bracing in a sitting position - Sit up in an alert and straight manner. While maintaining a steady breath, try pulling your navel inwards to touch your spine. It is not enough to imagine this procedure. You must carry it out.

Step 2: Channel energy to your muscles - As you hold your navel in, feel the muscles that are being employed in the process. While in this position and state of mind visualize yourself directing energy into your muscles from within you.

Step 3: Hold the position - If you are a beginner you can hold this position for a minimum of 30 seconds. However, the recommended time is five minutes. Always remember to keep breathing evenly.

As you continue with this exercise, you need to try to apply feelings of power, vibrant health and motivation to your body. This makes it easy to get the inspiration to match your visualization to your physical workouts. However, this is a technique that only works for small toning cases. For an overall toning of your body muscles you need proper exercising techniques you can combine with creative visualization. Furthermore, it you have an existing health problem, have your doctor check you up and get the relevant professional medication your body requires before you begin this exercise program.

c)   Use Creative Visualization to Look After your Heart

There are very many benefits you get when your heart is healthy. When you ensure your heart is in good condition you increase your blood flow and the distribution of oxygen all through your body. This lets you enjoy:

- High energy levels and increased endurance
- Low blood pressure
- Reduced body fat and a healthier body weight
- Less stress, anxiety and depression
- Better sleep

The best way to look after your heart is to engage in aerobics. This is an exercise that causes you to breathe deeply and make you sweat for a minimum of 20 minutes. Whether it is fast walking, swimming, jogging, biking or even cross-country skiing, you should be in a position to make a conversation.

How to Combine Aerobics with Creative Visualization

Step 1: Visualize your exercise activity – In your mind, visualize taking a 20-minute jog, fast walk or any other aerobic activity. You can visualize yourself wearing the right exercising clothes and suitable running shoes.

Step 2: Visualize yourself doing the activity – Here, you need to visualize how you feel in the training wear, how the running shoes fit your feet perfectly, the country lane or suburbs in which you are running through and start the exercise. Feel the power and strength in your feet and envision your arms moving back and forth to the rhythm of your legs feel the strength in your body and maintain your balance in a relaxed and simple position.

Step 3: Visualize yourself keeping pace for 20 minutes – In your mind's eye you can make yourself realize that although you are getting tired you are also energized and can well keep your pace until you are done. Imagine sweat building on your brow; you mop it away; your body feels supple and is moving easily to the finish line.

Step 4: Imagine the scenery – As you jog imagine passing trees, houses and you nod to people or wave at them. You should seem to enjoy the fact that they see you serious about your health. In your mind breath in and out, feel the refreshing coolness of the cool air and how refreshing it is to your lungs.

Step 5: Finish your exercise – You should continue your visualization exercise until you see yourself finish it. See yourself slowing down and returning to a normal walking pace and how your body feels fit and healthy.

While this visualization is still fresh in your mind plan to get yourself a jogging gear to do a 20 minutes aerobic exercise. After your first jog you will realize it is easy if you visualize the whole process and act it out as you exercise. You can do this exercise three times in a week or more if you can to maintain a healthy heart. Remember to consult your doctor if you have any health issues before you start any aerobic exercises. Additionally, if you feel the exercise is painful for you or you become short of breath you should stop.

d)   Use Creative Visualization to Build Stamina

For you to overcome all the challenges that come with changing bad habits you need to have both mental and physical stamina. This keeps you going and provides you the energy you need to overcome through the long haul. Your mental stamina helps you stick to your plans up to their completion. It is the physical stamina that provides you the energy you need to move your body through the whole process of your plans.

When using creative visualization to build your stamina you need breathing exercises. These exercises not only help you increase your stamina but also provide your body with the endurance you need to complete any activity you are engaged in. With the Chi breathing exercise your goal should be to relax your shoulders and chest by breathing deeply from within your abdomen.

- Hold your hands over your lower stomach and sit in an upright position
- Breathe deeply until you cannot draw in more air then let it all out to the last gasp
- Repeat this action more than once
- Visualize yourself breathing in with your hands sucking the air down all the way to your torso and into them
- Visualize yourself exhaling with your hands pushing air back through your stomach
- Slowly take your time settling into a slow, steady and comfortable rhythm
- Imagine the deep and continuing energy each breath you take brings to you

As you breathe in and out you should feel your abdomen expanding and contracting and the breathing moving all the way to your pelvic area. Practicing this exercise regularly is a good way to increase your endurance energy levels and build on your stamina level.

Chapter 6:
Meditation to Release Stress

With concerns regarding mental health arising, you will soon find that the major players such as **fear**, **despair**, and **negativity** all tend to stem from the same root factor - **stress**. Meditation has a wonderful ability to help in stress management. Not only does guided meditation allow you to help build your mental resilience, it is also an extremely effective tool to help relax your body and mind on a more immediate basis.

Stress relief meditation, in particular, can be used not only to help improve your mental state of being but also to help you release the physical tension you feel in your own body due to anxiety.

Meditative Guide to Help with Stress Relief

In this particular form of meditation, we will be dealing with finding a way for you to release your inner struggles, your worries, your sorrows, and your stress. To begin, you want to create a peaceful atmosphere around yourself. Surround yourself with dim lights, set your room to a comfortable temperature, and, if you choose, light a candle or set out essential oils to help bring forth a calming aura.

You Are Now Ready to Start Your Meditative Guide.

Before you close your eyes, look closely around you, and make a careful mental note of the things you see. Once you are done, close your eyes and focus on a fixed point in your mind's eye. Then, purge yourself of negativity and negative thoughts by carefully breathing into the count of five, holding your breath until the count of four, and then releasing to the count of three.

Breathe in.

Hold.

Release.

Breathe in.

Hold.

Release.

Breathe in.

Hold.

Release.

With your eyes closed, focus your mind on the sounds that you hear around you. Look past these sounds, and beyond them, you will find the voices of the people you love most dearly. Your loved ones and your well-wishers are all gathered here around you in a circle, amidst which you are seated.

The sounds you hear around you are slowly morphing into the voices of the people you love.

Breathe in.

Hold.

Release.

Focus on the voices – the voices are talking to you.

As you do so, start to identify the fears that are holding you in place. What scares you? What intimidates you? What do you fear?

Mentally assign a bold color to each of these fears and color them in so that you can see how strong their hold on you is.

Breathe in.

Hold.

Release.

See the colors swarm you and intertwine with the other – fear into insecurity, insecurity into greed, greed into falsehoods, and so on and so forth.

As you do start to focus on the voice once again, try to hear what they are saying.

Breathe in.

Hold.

Release.

Notice that they are reminding you of your worth.

You are good.

You are kind.

You are loved.

You are needed.

You are cherished.

You are wanted.

Breathe in.

Hold.

Release.

Every voice is manifesting in the form of a bright white light that is blasting through the bold reds, blues, and greens of your fears and is opening tiny breaks through which you can release yourself.

Breathe in.

Hold.

Release.

Remind yourself that the love and belief that they have in you is enough to set you free.

As you do this, travel through your body with your next breath and do so physically for yourself.

Breathe in.

As you feel the breath travel down through your shoulders, consciously let the tension loose, feel your shoulders flex backward, and release the weight on your shoulders as you allow the energy to flow through your entire being.

Each particle of energy is now changing from a chain to a bright searing white light which is radiating through your body.

Breathe in.

Hold.

Release.

Remind yourself of the things that are shifting inside of you as you feel the transformation take place.

You are calm and relaxed.

You are loved and respected.

You are letting go of all of the unwanted fears that hold you back and instead, you are filling yourself with stillness.

Breathe in.

Hold.

Release.

Remember that with each breath, you are releasing your concerns, and with each release, you are becoming lighter and lighter until you are but the weight of a feather adrift in the wind.

Repeat after me: I am supported and loved, and stressful situations do not scare me - they merely challenge me.

I am calm and centered, and calmness washes over me with every breath that I take.

Repeat it again, in your heart: I am supported and loved, and stressful situations do not scare me - they merely challenge me.

I am calm and centered, and calmness washes over me with every breath that I take.

Breathe in.

Hold.

Release.

As you slowly open your eyes, you will feel a physical burn shift from your shoulders and, instead of stress and pain, you will feel only thankfulness and courage.

Chapter 7:
Hypnosis and Meditation

We need to know about the hypnotherapy to understand weight loss hypnosis. Hypnosis is a technique in which therapists aim at calming people and helping them improve concentrate.

Many people find this methodology controversial, but it has been established that this procedure is authentic. When Hypnosis increases the internal concentration that a highly relaxed state produces, participants become more concentrated. This is when the subconscious mind is involved, and that portion of the consciousness is at ease.

Among physicians, hypnotherapy is conventional to help patients improve behaviors, manage anxiety and mood disorders, avoid depression, stop smoking, and alleviate pain. Besides, patients can also learn to support themselves and practice self-hypnosis.

Inspired by the promising outcomes of the successful hypnotherapy test, medical professionals are now investigating ways to use the effects of Hypnosis for weight loss.

During that phase, the subconscious mind of a patient is awakened. It is relevant because research shows that decision-making is affected by the subconscious mind. Therefore, when a person is hypnotized, what seems impossible or unachievable under normal circumstances becomes easy to solve.

Hypnosis allows patients to recognize critical areas that impede their progress and helps them to act determinedly on them. This is when patients can improve themselves without external pressure. They make better choices about food, avoid unhealthy habits and adopt a healthy routine. That is how hypnotherapy for weight loss aims to address the issue.

Hypnosis may also be primarily known as the party trick used to make some people do the chicken dancing on stage, but many people have turned to mind-control therapy to enable them to make healthier choices and lose weight—case by case.

Who Would Try Hypnosis?

Hypnosis is for those trying a gentle way to lose weight and make a habit of eating healthfully. For one guy, isn't it? Anyone wants a fast fix. This takes time to reframe negative feelings about food.

People's excuses struggle to lose weight.

1. **Missed inspiration:** Notwithstanding, seemingly every woman you meet complaining about her size and the shape – in fact most people are not serious about weight loss. The idea is that it is difficult to lose weight, will entail 'missing out' on foods you enjoy and will inevitably mean depriving yourself. This need not be the case with Hypnosis, the choice of how you change your behavior is entirely up to you as you are entirely in control of your actions through the power of your unconscious mind.

2.   **Unrealistic Goals:** Most of us just like the models and celebrities we see on TV and in magazines want to be the ideal size and form. Many people spend enormous amounts of energy, effort and resources in most situations – and could be blessed with significant genes too. We all want to look beautiful, slim and sexy, yeah, and please by the end of next week! And yet we are all of these things already – it is just that we forget sometimes. Weight loss is also about wanting to look healthy. Sometimes it is about feeling healthy. Hypnosis will also help you to understand your beauty and self-worth, and then build healthier behaviors to help you accomplish those things both within and outside!

3.   **Too early to give up:** We just want to be slim-now! As soon as a, b, or c diet doesn't work for us within two flat days, we give up. "For me, it didn't fit". And yet it has taken us several months, even years to build up the excess weight. Hypnosis takes place immediately. The moment you listen is the moment you start to change your mind and therefore alter your behavior, and then the outcome will inevitably change. And all right, maybe by the end of the week, you won't be 14lbs lighter – but I've seen tests from a 7lbs client in a week before now! Yeah, and she said it was the best thing she ever could have done! This is workable stuff.

4.   **Not Healthy Eating:** Most people can never get slim on chocolate, alcohol and fries because they're loaded with 'empty' calories that don't offer any nutritional value. The positive thing about these conventional diets is they allow you to eat healthy – lots of fruits, vegetables and foods that are naturally low in fats.

Hypnosis will help you make the right decisions for your loss of body, mind and weight – and yet let you enjoy the foods you love too!

5.   **Dieting not eating:** Over the past few decades, the billion-dollar diet industry has misled you. When you eat, you will not lose weight (long-term). Yeah, I know, that's controversial and is the topic for another post – but the fact remains that research has shown that only 2-3 per cent of people who lose weight on a diet can successfully hold the weight off in the long term.

You deprive yourself when you limit the consumption of food in any way by dieting. The mental deprivation comes from realizing that as soon as you know that everything you want more is not allowed – and finally give in and have it! The physical denial comes from knowing that you start eating it again as soon as you can eat it again (you come off the diet when you reach your goal) and the weight goes back straight on. Hypnosis will help you achieve healthy, positive and sustainable weight loss by modifying your food choices, eating habits and body image.

Why Can Hypnosis Aid Weight Loss?

Hypnosis is one of the best methods for weight loss, as it looks at the symptoms and tries to tackle the issue in its full depth. Hypnosis is not linked to calorie counting and the implementation of extreme restrictions. A therapist can get "access" to subconscious experiences and patterns of thought, making it easier to introduce new behaviors and process satisfaction.

Why, then, is Hypnosis such a great weight loss option?

1.   **Strong Reinforce.** The majority of weight loss plans are highly restrictive. They mention foods to avoid and those that will lead to weight gain. Those methods concentrate on negative feedback and patterns of restriction.

In comparison, Hypnosis provides constructive suggestions. After many sessions, you'll start enjoying nutritious foods and snacks even more than you used to.

2.   **Control Cravings.** Capability. Cravings are a significant factor for struggling to lose weight. Patients learn how to regulate these cravings by Hypnosis and how to make them vanish.

Good therapists may allow patients to 'give' away from the cravings during sessions. Since undergoing hypnotherapy, several people managed to keep their sugar and chocolate cravings under control.

3.   **Modification of habits.** Via Hypnosis, you will learn to enjoy foods that had been anything but enjoyable before. It's all about shifting the current subconscious habits which will offer you gratification. Junk food, candy, carbonated drinks or chocolate shakes may be implicated in these trends.

A hypnotherapist can focus on those responses being updated. You'll learn to settle for new vegetable juices and ice tea rather than carbonated drinks. "Learning" how to make the most of these safe choices eventually results in weight loss.

You cannot be compelled by a hypnotherapist to do anything you don't like.

Some people speak of Hypnosis as a misunderstanding. It possibly stems from the way Mass Media depicts hypnotherapy. As a result, individuals are worried that they will be pressured to do something they do not want or that will cause humiliation and shame for them.

In reality, Hypnosis is a deep relaxation state that makes you more open to suggestion and able to access memories or subconscious connections. To gain from hypnotherapy for weight loss, you just have to crave weight loss. The more driven you are, the faster the benefits you'll reap.

Today's world is just so fast-paced that it feels like we have no time to slow down, relax and be calm. Even when we go on holiday, we take over the office and work in our heads, worrying about the next board meeting, a disgruntled client, or where the next deal comes from.

We think we're happy and calm, but within our minds, there are many hidden stresses, fears, worries and thoughts going deep. When we don't take time to relax and quiet the inner noise consciously and intentionally, tension will build up and inevitably affect the quality of our lives, and how we deal with people around us.

It needn't be like this. Meditation practice will allow us to calm down and get still. It helps our mind to get concentrated and relax, helping us to cope with all the everyday stresses of a hectic life.

Not Just a Religious Act.

People typically classify meditation as being purely for religious or spiritual activities. Although many religions are correct to make meditation part of their religious practice, it is not merely a religious activity alone. But more and more people who aren't religious accept meditation practice.

If you feel like life is getting a little too hectic and leaving you stressed out, then slowing down, calming and relaxing would be a great time. Meditation will help you achieve the relaxed state you need to ease your mind and free from stress.

Meditative Advantages.

Still, wondered why people are meditating? Which difference, which value does it bring to their lives? I was at a low point in my life when I started meditating and crying about the loss of my friend. I started meditating on my counsellor's suggestions as a way to help ease my worries and continue my wellbeing and core strength building cycle.

A lot of people have various reasons to meditate. When you are contemplating, what was your reason to meditate? To an outsider, if you meditate what they see you do is sit down, maybe cross-legged on the floor, staring at a point in the distance or sit with your eyes closed.

How does this, practicing meditation, influence your state of mind? Yet most of my students in yoga and meditation swear that meditation for 15 minutes a day is the best thing they can do to give them the strength, motivation and compassion they need to do whatever they need.

Meditation is some mental activity that has significant health benefits both for the mind and the body. Meditation can help relax the mind, establish a more concentrated state and enhance the functioning of the brain.

Medical evidence suggests that meditation practice appears to elicit a level of physiological relaxation: decreases in blood pressure, slower heartbeats and faster breathing, and other biochemical improvements can occur as well.

Chapter 8:
What is a Gastric Band?

The gastric band (also known as a lap band) has become an increasingly popular surgical procedure for those who want to lose weight during the last decade or so. A band is fitted around the stomach and inflated in a way that significantly decreases stomach ability. This means the patient consumes less food, which leads to a fast and lasting weight loss.

But surgery with the gastric band isn't without complications. With any surgery of something going wrong, there's always the inherent risk, but there are also some issues that the lap band can specifically cause. It involves a slipped band (which can result in too much or not enough stomach capacity), acid reflux, nausea, vomiting, diarrhea, regurgitation, blockages and other problems. And although the findings are unquestionably impressive, there are definitely hidden risks. But wouldn't it be awesome if there had been a way of replicating the gastric band's success without any of the risks?

Yeah, there's definitely away in there. Recently hypnotherapists repeated the lap band treatment solely with hypnotic suggestions with great results. No scalpels, anesthetics, or wounds-pure mind-power. Hypnotherapy has become the latest craze in weight loss due to its safe and impacts the existence of the gastric band. A quick search on Google shows hundreds of happy patients who have undergone hypnotherapy in the gastric band and lost much of their excess weight. But how exactly does it work?

To understand how gastric band hypnotherapy functions, first, we need to look at hypnosis and the mental effect. Although human mental awareness is far from complete, the most welcoming theory is that the mind consists of two major components-the conscious and the subconscious. You should be most familiar with the idea of conscious thinking because this is from where the daily cycle of thought originates. Whenever you think to yourself, "I am thirsty, I should go get a drink" or something similar that is at work in your conscious mind. Your subconscious mind is much deeper and, in a way, stronger. It governs all those instinctive behaviors and responses you're not really thinking about, your routines, your impulses, and your phobias. Hypnosis operates upon the subconscious mind. The subconscious is primed by hypnosis and able to consider suggestions.

Now we understand how hypnosis works; it is a little clearer how hypnotherapy works on the gastric unit. A hypnotherapist can create a hypnotic state within their client and then speak to them as if it were really occurring via the gastric band technique. There is no pain or something really happening physically at all, but it is very difficult for the subconscious mind to distinguish between illusion and reality. This is why very strong dreams can often seem all too real.

If the subconscious mind assumes that the body is fitted with a gastric band, it will behave as though you are fitted with one. That means you'll feel full faster, eat slowly, and consume smaller meals. This obviously results in weight loss, which is very important.

In addition to being safer than surgery, hypnotherapy by the gastric band is also much more convenient-generally ten times less costly than surgery. There are also professional hypnotherapists selling audio packs that have the very same session on CD or MP3 that are even less costly because the hypnotherapist only has to record the session once with certain clients. It will cost inferior to $100.

And if you are thinking of getting surgery with the gastric band, then the normal form of hypnotherapy might well be worth your consideration.

Hypnotherapy Gastric Band Hypnosis

If you're clinically obese-BMI over 30-there's hope with a virtual gastric band placed under hypnosis-sure, hypnotherapy may be the best all-round weight-loss choice.

I have run two successful tandem weight loss programs and so have had great experience supporting other people with their weight issues-both programs have the same philosophies at their heart. Many people on a diet are eating the items they shouldn't eat or go back to their old ways after dieting and losing weight. Some of their diets that exclude certain foods-leaving an unbalanced diet that puts a strain on their liver and kidneys-which are potentially very dangerous.

I think it's important to get people in touch with the joy of eating healthy food and persuade them of the cost-effectiveness of consuming less good quality food rather than cheaper fat sugar and salt-saturated foods-good nutrition really provides greater value for the buck, and after all, you wouldn't put paraffin in your fuel tank? You wouldn't put fuel in the car to take the metaphor further for comfort eaters if the oil light comes on, would you? Yet the oil light is a sign that something is wrong and putting chocolate in your mouth won't fix the problems. Comfort food fixes little but gives rise to obesity.

Some of these issues are related to anxiety tension or lack of self-confidence or childhood behaviors rooted in bad eating practices as they grew up: "you have to clear your plate"-for example. I say pounds more in the waste bin than pounds on the floor!

Hypnotherapy may tackle these concerns-providing approaches to cope with anxiety and depression and loss of confidence and using methods such as regression to cope with psychological issues that could have contributed to an unhealthy relationship with food. One lady of 21 stones came to me, and after we had dealt with her bullying problems and offered her dietary advice, she immediately started to lose weight-something she should never have done!

Furthermore, the American Health Authority also blames a lot of obesity on fast food-which you can also call "junkie" food-the food has added fat sugar and salt, and the taste buds are actually addicted to this stuff-if you've ever seen "Supersize me" you know how unhealthy it can be, especially if the eating style is skewed to junk food.

The food diary is another valuable tool-to remember what you eat but also when and why you consume those foods?

When obesity hits a BMI point of over 30 then for some the option is strong: if they don't lose weight, they'll have serious health problems-they'll have tried all the diets and pills and found them to fail because they haven't solved any of the underlying reasons for overeating. Often they are left with a Gastric Band's only option-the the operation will cost about £3,000-£ 7,000-in some situations the operation can be risky-I just had a client who had several strokes and two of them extreme-the risks are too great for her.

Combining good nutritional advice with learning to properly enjoy food and dealing with underlying psychological problems can result in permanent weight loss. Alternatively, putting the Virtual Gastric band under hypnosis, using something called the Hypogastric Band system, makes weight loss even more probable. The machine works with most people, and consumers have mentioned not only being able to see and observe the procedure without discomfort but also being able to feel it when it's installed. The discomfort passes quickly, and people find that they start eating smaller portions and, like my other customers who lose weight, they eat less and exercise more and start enjoying the food again.

The procedure of the gastric band is spoken about under hypnosis, and because it is keyhole surgery it is relatively easy-wrapping a band around the higher part of the stomach-the band can be tightened or loosened, and the golf ball-sized portion of the stomach created by the band means that the hypothalamus, the appetite regulator, informs you that you are complete-the food passes about naturally. The hypnotic stomach band placed under hypnosis works the same way as a real stomach band. There are also weight reduction plans that do the same but skip wearing the gastric band if you have a BMI under 30.

And if you have tried the others and it has failed, try hypnotherapy. My experience is, it's a practical option for most people.

Do Hypnosis Gastric Bands Really Work?

Lately, there's been a lot of press reports about the virtual hypnotic gastric band, but does that work? The vast quantity of websites out there would have you believe it works, and it is successful.

Such websites will just tell you what they want you to know and will not show you the absolute truth. Yeah, there have been reports in the press, but are they not just press releases sent to their publications to improve this procedure's credibility?

There won't be any newspaper publishing an article saying the hypnotic gastric band doesn't work, so who will read it? It would be as if they were writing an article stating that children do not like eating vegetables; no one would read it. But if they released an article that says a new technique was discovered that would make kids enjoy vegetables, then it would be a different story.

Since this technique was on the market, there were no scientifically validated studies demonstrating the effectiveness of the virtual hypnotic gastric unit.

This weight-loss strategy is no different from the conventional weight-loss methods that want you to believe they have the solution to your weight problem. We want you to believe their treatment will instantly turn off the mental and physiological factors that generate the weight issue right now. No treatment can do that, particularly if it doesn't tackle the real reasons why you're having a weight issue.

Having done one of those procedures is just like cutting off the head of a plant. At first, you think it's gone, and you start making progress, but those roots begin to crave the light underground. Then gradually, they start breaking the surface of the soil, at which point the old patterns of actions begin to take over again. You could then say to yourself that you deserve this chocolate bar because you were so good. Finally, those weeds start flowering and start taking up more of your lawn, at which point you give up trying to lose weight completely.

The hypnotic band may help some people temporarily lose weight, but over time people may start stretching out the limits of this procedure, as some do with the actual surgical version. The one thing about overeating mental and physiological factors is that if they aren't treated, they will come back again. This may be during one of those times a person undergoes emotional stress. The person can then use the food as a comfort either consciously or even unconsciously.

The individual then goes back to believing after this event that they have a gastric band fitted but that one little slip up has now undermined the confidence. The next time the person goes through some emotional stress, then it's even easier for them to use food for comfort because they've done it in the past already.

Chapter 9:
Strong Hypnotic Gastric Band - The Weekly Program.

Practice regularly, self-hypnosis helps relieve stress, anxiety, physical pain. The first step: learn to relax your mind. Suggested by Lise Bartoli, psychologist, and hypnotherapist, these three self-hypnosis exercises will help you.

Autonomous, they can then evolve by themselves". Its program consists of several phases. Here, we'll only cover the first - major - step of learning to relax. But first, some tips for successful exercises.

Choose the right time. You can test different schedules. Either early in the morning, early evening, or on weekends.

A word of advice: better avoid self-hypnosis sessions late in the evening, you might fall asleep. Plan a quiet beach. Before each exercise, make sure you are not disturbed and turn off the ringer on your phone. Even if the duration of the exercises depends on each one, allow 30 to 45 minutes of availability.

Choose the right place. At home, test several places until you find the one where you feel really good to land. Once chosen, you will always put yourself in the same place when you practice a self-hypnosis session.

Make yourself comfortable. Wear loose clothing and sit in a comfortable seat with your head properly seated for optimal relaxation. Avoid the lying position, which promotes sleep.

Memorize the course of the exercise or register. If it's easier to relax by letting yourself be guided, record yourself reading the text of the statement. Speak in a monotone voice while articulating carefully. Leave breaks long enough to have time to respond to instructions.

Evolve at your own pace. Those who are used to relaxing can do all three exercises in a row. For the others, it will be better to repeat each of them until it is fluid, then move on to the next day.

Monday   Self Hypnosis Motivation to Lose Weight

Step by Step to Lose Weight with Hypnosis

Losing weight with hypnosis works just like any other change with hypnosis will. However, it is important to understand the step by step process so that you know exactly what to expect during your weight loss journey with the support of hypnosis. In general, there are about seven steps that are involved with weight loss using hypnosis.

- The first step is when you decide to change
- The second step involves your sessions
- The third and fourth are your changed mindset and behaviors
- The fifth step involves your regressions
- The sixth is your management routines

- The seventh is your lasting change.

To give you a better idea of what each of these parts of your journey looks like, let us explore them in greater detail below.

In your first step toward achieving weight loss with hypnosis, you have to decide that you desire change and that you are willing to try hypnosis to change your approach to weight loss. At this point, you know you want to lose weight, and you have been shown the possibility of losing weight through hypnosis. You may find yourself feeling curious, open to trying something new, and a little bit skeptical as to whether this is actually going to work for you. You may also be feeling frustrated, overwhelmed, or even defeated by the lack of success you have seen using other weight loss methods, which may be what lead you to seek out hypnosis in the first place. At this stage, the best thing you can do is practice keeping an open and curious mind, as this is how you can set yourself up for success when it comes to your actual hypnosis sessions.

Your sessions account for stage two of the process. Technically, you are going to move from stage two through to stage five several times over before you officially move into stage six. Your sessions are the stage where you engage in hypnosis, nothing more, and nothing less. During your sessions, you need to maintain your open mind and stay focused on how hypnosis can help you. If you are struggling to stay open-minded or are still skeptical about how this might work, you can consider switching from absolute confidence that it will help to have a curiosity about how it might help instead.

Following your sessions, you are first going to experience a changed mindset. This is where you start to feel far more confident in your ability to lose weight and in your ability to keep the weight off. At first, your mindset may still be shadowed by doubt, but as you continue to use hypnosis and see your results, you will realize that you can create success with hypnosis. As these pieces of evidence start to show up in your own life, you will find your hypnosis sessions becoming even more powerful and even more successful.

In addition to a changed mindset, you are going to start to see changed behaviors.

Tuesday   Self Hypnosis to overcome Compulsive/Emotional Eating

The "resource place."

Now imagine a place of relaxation that will deeply relax you.

Let your unconscious make you discover the images of a place of nature, which is for your symbol of harmony and well-being. It can be a known or imaginary place, whatever. The main thing is that you feel good in this place: whether it is a sandy beach, a corner of the countryside or a green mountain.

Look around, perceive what it is possible to feel (the sound of the waves, the blue of the sky, the smell of flowers, and the song of birds). The many sensory details developed mentally are important, because they allow you to build a place of your own, your own, a unique place of which you will feel creative.

Stay there as long as you want. You can lie down or take a walk.

Wednesday   Rest

Thursday   Self Hypnosis Motivation to Lose Weight

Interior light once plunged into the state of calm induced by the preceding exercise, continue by visualizing a soft color: blue, golden, and orange.

Imagine that the color you have chosen emanates from the earth and then goes up to you. It enters your whole body, starting with the feet. It relaxes each muscle.

The feet relax. Now bring the light up to the top of your head and enjoy this moment of relaxation. Focusing on a soft interior color leads to a number of physiological changes: lower blood pressure, slower breathing, and an even greater inner feeling of calm.

Friday   Self Hypnosis Motivation to Lose Weight

Here and Now Sit comfortably and choose a fixed point in front of you. It can be a painting or any other object.

While fixing this point, mentally check all the parts of your body by listing your perceptions: "I hear the rumor of the city," "I feel the warmth of the wood of the chair under my palms" ... Listening to your sensations, you will gradually relax your alertness.

Fix the point until your eyelids tend to close on their own. Then continue to detail your sensations with your eyes closed. Then focus your attention on the air that you breathe, and that goes to your lungs, then guide it towards your belly. The latter inflates like a balloon and brings you more lightness. As you practice this breathing, you will feel your body becoming lighter and lighter. Savor this moment of tranquility and calm.

Saturday   Self Hypnosis for Sense of Satiety

After becoming familiar with self-hypnosis and gaining confidence, you will go into self-hypnosis, and you then ask yourself and make the most of all the bites of this much-desired food.

It starts with the eyes, you touch it with your lips, you feel it, you touch it with your tongue, you feel it in your mouth, you taste it, you breathe it, and it all happens in full consciousness, focusing on every sensation.

Then you swallow the bite, and then you open your eyes. To look again at your favorite food and wonder if you still want it. If so, then you start the self-hypnosis exercise again. All this happens slowly; in the rhythm proper to Hypnosis, and in a unique perception of the food, nothing exists anymore.

Sunday   Rest

Chapter 10:
Healing Yourself – Relaxation Techniques

Every human has their methods of relaxing, which can be unique and different from the general method others relax. However, relaxation is an essential part of our lives that we must not neglect. There are various relaxation methods, ranging from simple and easy techniques to complex techniques. So, you need to find the most suitable technique for you.

Tips to Relaxation

Relaxation is a very simple process, which is achieved by any means, yet you need a guide on how to achieve relaxation.

- Don't be too hard on yourself when you are trying to relax. Any relaxation method is to help you relax both your body and mind.
- Your environment must be quiet and free from distractions.
- Your position must be comfortable, whether sitting or lying
- Relax over few minutes firstly
- Have a routine of relaxation
- Be consistent
- Relaxation Technique
- Progressive muscle relaxation
- This simple means flexing, tightening and relaxing your muscles by progression. You tense and then release these

muscle groups one by one. Examples, you tense and relax the muscles in the face first and which you move to the muscles in your hands, and arms. Another form of progressive muscle relaxation is passive muscle relaxation. You do not need to tighten or make the already tighten muscles tight any longer. You just need to release and relax your muscles from the beginning of the technique.

- Imagery meditation or visualization help to relax your body and mind through the use of pictures
- Relaxation hypnosis
- Autogenic relaxation is the ability to imagine that some of your body parts, limbs especially.
- Other techniques include exercise, the use of the sensory organs to get relaxed. Deep breathing exercises and;
- Knowing which relaxation technique works for you is to try them at least.
- Relaxation Process
- Relaxation Hypnosis is a sate whereby you enter into a great level of relaxation, by first quieting your conscious mind and allowing your sub-consciousness to dominate more.
- Begin to have a good feeling all over your body as you sit in a comfortable position.
- You feel every nerve and muscle in your body is getting loose, and you are becoming relaxed
- You feel your arms getting relaxed and light

- This is a good feeling, and you are getting more relaxed gradually
- You feel a great sensation all over your body, from your head to your toes
- Let your muscle feel released and loose
- You begin to feel more relaxed, as you take each breath
- You begin to feel sleepy as you breathe in and out
- Deeper and calmer, you continue breathing in and out
- You are feeling very relaxed, and your muscles are loosed
- Your arm is getting lighter and relaxed. More relaxed as you hear your silent heartbeat.
- You are calmer as you breathe in and out, drowsier and sleepier.
- Progressive Muscle
- This exercise is to help you relax the muscles of your body. You will be asked to tighten your muscles and release them during this technique.
- Stay in a comfortable position, adjust until you feel really comfortable and the position is painless
- Close your eyes when you are ready, and breathe in through your nose. Take a deep breath, then hold your breath for a few seconds, and then exhale slowly.
- You begin to feel relaxed, at this point
- Hold your breath, and then let go
- Allow yourself to become more relaxed
- Now, tilt your forehead, and raise your eyes up as though you are looking at the sky

- Raise your forehead, and you begin to feel tense, and tightened in your neck and head.
- You begin to feel relaxed
- Focus on your forehead, and now relax your forehead and notice the way you feel
- As you feel tension, you feel your mind wandering around, and you feel like relaxed now
- Let all the tension drain and let go from you
- Let your eyes, nose, and face feel tensed, and focus on it.
- Begin to feel relaxed
- Breath in and out
- You feel relaxed, focus more relaxing
- Notice your mind becoming relaxed
- Now, focus on your jaw and smile widely. You feel your teeth clenched to each other, and now relax those muscles
- Relax your face and notice the feeling that comes from relaxation
- You feel comfortable, as your face and jaw become more and more released
- Relax your face little more
- Breathe in deeply, hold your breath and breathe out
- Release your muscles and let go of your muscle
- Tense the muscles around your back, neck, and shoulders, but shrugging your shoulders and turning your neck
- Tilt your neck, and feel the tension around your neck loosing up

- Then move to your shoulders. Try to lift your shoulders to touch your ears, feel the tension in your shoulders and neck released and now let go of these muscles
- Feel your shoulders becoming more comfortable
- Move your arms, and hold your hands together, raising your hands towards your shoulders. You begin to feel released and relaxed.
- Take a deep breath and then let go
- You feel the tension flow out of your shoulders, arms, and hands
- Relax your arms, hands, and shoulders.
- Now, focus on your breathing and abdominal muscles
- Take another deep breath through your nose
- Breathe in and out
- Feel the rising in your chest as you breathe out
- Repeat the action, breathe in through your nose, hold your breath and let go
- Notice the free relaxation you feel as you breathe out
- Feel the relaxation around our abdomen that has spread across your face, your hands, arms, and neck
- Relax as far as you can
- You feel as if you have a soft pillow behind your back, and you feel deeply relaxed
- Shift your focus on your shoulder, as though you want it to fall apart from your body towards your spine.
- Make your shoulders feel tensed, and let go now
- Let the relaxation spread into every muscle of your back

- Feel relaxed
- Take a breath in and out
- You begin to feel every pain in your back becoming released
- Go deeper into relaxing these muscles, and now tighten your abdomen
- Hold this position and now relax
- Soften your abdomen, feel your belly becoming more relaxed
- Relaxation is spreading across every part of your abdomen
- Tighten your lower limbs, the hips, thighs and down to your feet,
- Begin from your hips, feel the tension in your hips and release it now
- Take another deep breath and focus on your hips and thighs
- You begin to feel relaxed, and the tension in your hips is becoming released
- Then focus on your thigh, you feel it tensed, let go now
- You feel relieved, and the tension is released in your thigh
- Place your hands and your thigh and feel them becoming relaxed and softened
- Then move to your knee, at this point you feel tighten in your knees, let go of the tightened
- Focus on the relaxation
- You feel blood and oxygen rushing through your knees
- Release the knees and take another deep breath
- Let the relaxation spread deeper from your hips o your knees
- Now, we move to your toes and knees. Feel the tension in your toes and then feet

- Release your feet and toes, and you feel relaxed
- Move back to the ankle of your legs, try to turn your legs around
- Tighten the ankle for few seconds and let it go
- You feel the tension becoming released
- You feel more released, as you feel the relaxation spreading across your feet, toes, and ankles
- Feel the sense of reliving in your body as the tension is being released. Enjoy this relaxation
- Scan your entire body, allow your awareness focus on each part of your body and let every remaining tension be taken care of
- Scan your forehead, relax and feel released, move to your face, eyes, nose, and mouth and let go of every tension
- Breathe in and out slowly
- Continue through every part of your body, your neck shoulders, chest, hands relaxed and released every tension
- Then your back, hips, abdomen, let go of every tension in the parts
- Then your knees, thigh, and toes, feel the tension in your body all wiped and flushed out of your body from your head to your toes
- Take a slow deep breath

Autogenic Relaxation

The autogenic relaxation technique involves generating relaxation within yourself and the body. The technique involves the individual relaxed, by imagining their body is warm and heavy.

This technique is to help your body feel warm and relaxed. And these are the steps

- Find a comfortable position, you may choose to sit or lie.
- Get settled into this position and try to notice the way your body. Simple notice the state of your body, and do not try to change anything.
- Take a deep breath, in and out
- Continue to take your breathing slowly
- Begin to imagine your body becoming relaxed in the tensed areas
- Focus your attention on your feet, and get relaxed. Your feet are getting more relaxed now and warm, from the top of your feet to the sole of your feet
- Shift your attention to your right foot, feel the top and sole of your foot.
- By now, you begin to feel a sensation of warmth and heaviness together in your feet, and the sensation begins to increase deeply.
- This sensation moves down to your ankles and legs and spreads across your toes; by now, you are more relaxed than the beginning of the technique.
- Shift your attention from your legs to your hands
- Focus on your right hand; feel the warmth spreading across your fingers and thumb, which is spreading across both of your palms.

- Focus on your left hand, too, feel the warmth spreading across the fingers, to the thumb, and to the palm.
- By now, your both hands are completely warm, heavy and relaxed
- The warmth spreads across to your wrist, and lower arms.
- You feel the sensation around your elbow, upper arms, wrists, and shoulders.
- You begin to feel deeply relaxed, and these parts feel heavy and very warm.
- Shift your attention to your feet and legs, you begin to feel warmth in your feet and legs, and this warmth is spreading across your lower legs, to the knees, joints, upper legs, thighs, and then to your joint.

Chapter 11:
Maintaining a Strong Daily Practice

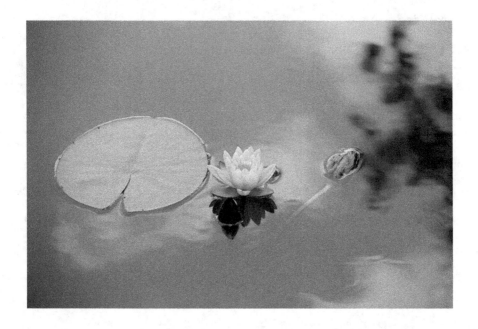

For your quick workout routine, walk up through the stairs at the office. Park your car at the farthest spot and trek all the way distance. Take your dog on a long walk. Participate in every way you can. That is the goal of exercising. If you miss any workout or you couldn't get going one day, don't just hang up on it, just get back on track the next day.

Set a routine for everyday hypnosis meditation and affirmation for weight loss

If you are stuck in the same old aerobics' classes, then you could mix things up and try to take a new class at your gym. Some of the hottest gym classes that you could take include indoor cycling, boxing based programs, yoga classes acrobatics, and martial art. This will help you to be able to combat boredom, which is the number one reason why you participate in emotional eating and quit exercising. Try always to drink a lot of water while exercising. Warm-up before exercising. If you haven't warmed up, then you have to get into the habit of warming up before every exercise. Make it a habit to warm up. It isn't necessary to warm up before any strenuous exercise, but by doing so, you'll be able to get your blood flowing, and you be able to prepare yourself for any activity ahead.

Standing Reach Stretch

One of the stretching exercises that you can do is the standing reach stretch. This stretch involves the upper body's movement. So start with your arms, keep your arms straight down, besides your body is with your palms facing backward. Use one arm, raise it forward, and raise it up as high as possible. Now tighten your abs and use the opposite arm to touch your shoulders and stretch across your chest slightly. Now hold the stretch for 10 to 30 seconds.

Repeat the same stretch with your arms reaching in the opposite direction. The neck stretches the chest and backstretch. Use your hands to grab the ends of a small towel in both hands. Now bring your arms to the chest level and slightly tuck on the ends of the towel and hold it for about 10 to 30 seconds.

Neck Stretch

Neck stretch is the upper body stretch. This stretch is very good for golfers. Grab the end of a small towel with your end and slightly tuck them to the end of the wall.

The chest and Shoulders stretch

Now the next stretch is the chest and shoulder stretch. This stretch is great after swimming. So, take your hands behind you, and hold the end of a towel at your hip. Now raise your chest high and raise your arms forward now hold the stretch for about 30 seconds.

Quadriceps Stretch

The next stretch is the quadriceps stretch. This stretch is good for runners, high-cut cyclists, and walkers. Sit behind the chair and hold onto the chair for balance and support. Now take one hand and grab your other ankle. Gently push your foot forward towards your gluts. Do not tuck or lean forward but keep your chest lifted high. Now do this stretch for about 10 to 30 seconds. Now repeat the same thing using the other leg.

Standing outer thigh stretch

Stand behind the chair and hold onto the back of the chair for balance. Place one of your feet behind the chair and diagonally press your heels to the floor. Hold the stretch for about 30 seconds and put it doing using your other leg.

Tendon Stretch Arm's Length

The next stretch is the tendon stretch stand. Keep your arm's length behind the chair and hold onto the back of the chair to support and balance yourself. Now keep your feet a few inches apart from your toes why you point your heels to the ground. Slowly push your pelvis while bending your elbows and leaning forward. Support yourself with your hands to the back of the chair. Now do this for about 30 seconds.

Standing thin stretch stand

The next stretch the standing shin stretch. Stand at the back of a chair and hold the back of the chair for support and balance. Bend your nails slightly and raise the toes of your feet off the ground while resting on your heels. Do this stretch for about 30 seconds.

Hip Stretch

The next one is the hip stretch. Stand at the back of a chair for support and balance while bending your nails across and cross one ankle over the opposite leg. Now sit back watch and hold it straight for about 30 seconds. Repeat the stretch, crossing the other ankle over the opposite knee.

Upper back Stretch and shoulder stretch

The next one is upper backstretch and shoulder stretch. This stretch is perfect for activities that require the upper body and bending movements. So, to begin the stretch, stand behind the chair and hold onto the back of the chair for support. Then take one step away from the chair until your arms are fully stretched. Now move and bend forward from your waist and stretch your shoulders forward, then hold onto the knee for about 30 seconds.

Try to stretch as many ways as you can; the more stretches that you do, the more likely, you will be to avoid tight muscles, prevent injuries, and feel better if your muscles are tight, patient with it. It will take some time for your muscles to go back to their normal length. Stretching throughout your life will help to reduce the effect of aging and will help me to lose weight and reduce the wear and tear of your joints and tissue.

 Studies have shown that it is possible to maintain your flexibility through a wide-stretching program that you can follow. You should remember that stretching is not a contest, you shouldn't compare yourself with other people because everybody is different. Some days you might be feeling bar where are some days you might feel tighter. Stay comfortably within your limits and allow the flow of your energy to come through you.

Now let us look talk about some simple exercises that will help you during your hypothesis session.

Abs

 The first one is the abs. So grab a bubble chair or a dumbbell and then lay your back on it while pointing your feet straight. Take the weight and extend your arms over it, and then contract your abdominal muscles while lifting the weight up towards the ceiling. Exhale while moving up and inhale while moving downward. Now you should remember not to bounce on the ball. Moves slowly so that your muscles will be tight throughout the entire set also try to bring your weight at an angle and try to push the weight straight all perfectly vertical. Now the equipment that you need for this exercise are dumbbells and exercise balls, whereas the muscles that you are working out are the upper abdominal and the core muscles.

Chapter 12:

Believe

The Vital Ingredients: Motivation, Belief, and Expectation

You command the vital ingredients which make self-hypnosis function for you. These are the very same ingredients that produce your experience of achievement for virtually any goal you select. Let's take a look at every element and the way you can use it to do for you.

Motivation

Success is the power of your appetite; of everything you would like. Needing is a sense which you're able to control. For most of your life, you've controlled mainly your appetite or needing by restricting it or denying it. You could be rather good at controlling your desires and needing certain regions and weak or unpracticed others. Since this is a "diet" book, you Might Have already prepared to listen to that this "diet" would probably be similar to others who have informed you what you have to deny limit or yourself. In other words, other diets also have told you precisely what not to desire, and the accent might have been about "not needing" a few foods you have grown to appreciate. Welcome to a different method of treating yourself; we will invite you to get better in "wanting."

Your motivation is an integral variable, among the fundamental and fundamental ingredients. We would like you to concentrate your energy of needing not toward food; however, toward the motivation which informs your mind-body everything you would like it to make ideal weight. We invite you to get great at wanting your ideal weight. Here's a good illustration. Let's suppose that you're in a pool and you breathe in a mouthful of water. In that instant, you need just one item, a breath of air. It seems just like life or death, and a breath of all atmosphere is the one thing on your head currently. The needing is so powerful and intense that it overshadows the rest of the ideas and propels one to do anything is required to find that breathe of air. That's just how much we would like you to need the exact burden and body image which you want.

Belief and Thinking

Beliefs are such ideas and ideas which are accurate for you. They don't need to be scientifically demonstrated that you understand them to be authentic for you. Whether you're conscious of it or not, your activities, both unconscious and conscious, are according to your own beliefs. Even though your beliefs come in the shape of ideas and thoughts, they form your expertise by changing your activities in life. If you feel that animals make fantastic companions, then you most likely have a dog or cat or parrot or a ferret or two. If you feel that coffee keeps you awake during the night, then you most likely don't drink coffee before going to bed.

The ability of thinking enables you to affect your entire body in a way which may appear astonishing. Placebo answers, where folks respond to an inert chemical as if it had been the right medicine, are typical examples of the way that beliefs have been experienced within the entire body. If an individual believes he will become well when carrying a specific medicine, it is going to take place if the pill includes drugs or is only perceptible. In precisely the same manner, if an individual believes he can attain high levels in school, it is going to occur.

If an individual believes he can reach his ideal weight, then it is going to occur. Recall your chosen matches as a kid. Your capacity to feign is equally as powerful now as if you're young. It Might Be a little rusty, and you may require a bit of exercise, but when you allow yourself to feign and let's think in what you're pretending, you are going to see a powerful instrument.

You will find that this can be a superbly productive method to produce your aims, these messages of everything you would like, to everyone the cells and organs and tissues of the human body, which react by bringing that aim in reality for you. We cannot state this enough: ideas are things. The ideas, the images, the thoughts which you set in your head become the messages that your self-hypnosis communicates into a mind-body, finally turning your ideal body to a truth. Pretending is picking what to think and getting absorbed in these thoughts. As a magnifying glass may concentrate beams of the sun, you can concentrate your emotional energy to create your ideas, thoughts, and beliefs actual for your physique.

Expectation

You might not always get what you would like, but you do get what you expect. Expectations include the power of faith, and eventually, become the outcomes of what's considered. Here's a good illustration of how to "expect." Once you sat down to read this novel, you didn't analyze the seat or couch to check its ability to maintain your weight. You simply sat down without even considering it.

You did not have to Consider It, because a piece of your convinced, and contains so much religion in the seat, which you "anticipated" it to maintain you. That's the best way to anticipate the ideal body weight you would like. Bearing this in mind, be cautious of everything you say to yourself and others seeing your body weight expectations. "I gain weight through the holidays" "Last evening I ate two pieces of cake, and this morning I had been just two pounds heavier."

Mind-Body in Focus

Every one of the vital ingredients may create powerful results when concentrated inside the mind-body. But when these ingredients have been calibrated correctly inside the procedure for self-hypnosis, their efficacy has still magnified a hundredfold. Self-hypnosis is a procedure for making your reality. You may think that sounds magic or too fantastic to be correct, but that's relative to what you've gotten up to this stage in your life. These thoughts may be quite fresh for you. Here's a good instance of this "comparative" character of fresh thoughts.

Imagine that you're supplied a personal jet that's beautifully equipped with luxury appointments and also a well-trained crew. It's a fantastic gift, and you also get to reveal this technology marvel to some people who have not ever seen anything like this. Let's suppose your pilot strikes you back in time to before December 17, 1903, when the Wright brothers declared their first flight in Kitty Hawk. You're happy to reveal this miracle of technology into the Wright brothers that are come to greet you personally. What could happen? Maybe they'd be scared and would not think it is possible to fly into a metallic bird. You can give them a ride, and they may opt to run out of you. Folks can reject or resist new ideas, even if they're lovely.

Stretch your perspective and allow yourself the chance to get knowledgeable about the thoughts of self-hypnosis. From the Quick weight loss diet, we're offering you thoughts that may extend your creativity and shrink your clothes size. To mention that self-hypnosis is a procedure where you make your reality might appear too fantastic to be accurate or perhaps incredible at this time, possibly as amazing as a time system is to get a few. That's nice, for now; a however open mind and creativity to the possibilities this provides you to achieve your ideal body weight. Let's believe this course of action is genuine and accurate, since it's, and since it depends upon your view to become authentic.

Your subconscious (mind-body) utilizes the combo of everything you need (inspiration), everything you think, and what you anticipate as a blueprint for actions. The outcomes are attained by your mind-body (unconscious), rather than by studying or thinking. If somebody reaches a cold surface, she thinks is quite sexy, she can generate a blister or burn reaction. Conversely, an individual touching a scorching surface, believing it is cold might not create a burn reaction. Individuals who walk across hot flashes while imagining they are cool might undergo thermal harm (some slight scorching around the bottoms of the feet); however, their immune system doesn't react with a burn (blistering, pain, etc.) since their heads inform their bodies the way to respond. Again, it's the orientation of three of those vital ingredients which makes it easy:

- desiring to take action
- thinking it possible
- hoping to become successful

The truth goes through three phases. First, it's ridiculed. Second, it's violently opposed. Third, it's considered to be self-evident.

That is the trick to achievement. Your entire body carries your own beliefs. Your beliefs guide your activities, which then form your expertise. Some explain this procedure as creating your achievement or producing your expertise in life.

In our civilization, we view this clarified within the inspirational and positive emotional attitude literature. It may be understood in several regions of metaphysics. It is also possible to look back to the ancients and watch that is explained in the details of the historic period.

An individual much wiser than we're mentioned, "It'll be done unto you based on your view." At the current era of integrative psychology and medicine, we predict it self-hypnosis or mind-body medication. There continue to be many scientific studies which demonstrate surprising consequences for pain management, wound healing, physical change, and a lot more health benefits than we thought possible.

Choosing Your Beliefs

You can pick your beliefs. You might decide to think what you find, in the feeling of "See it to believe it" or even "Seeing is believing" That is pretty simple to accomplish. You encounter something together with your perceptions, and that's a comfortable manner of picking whether it's believable or not. However, you might also opt to think about it and then watch it, which might require some exercise. Many men and women find it simpler to allow the world to tell them what's accurate or what to think. The T.V, newspapers, media, novels, teachers, and specialists bombard us with everything to think. You grew up learning about the planet and yourself from several outside resources. It also led to a recognizable routine of discovering and observing information concerning the planet from yourself, and you decided which advice to create part of your belief system.

It comprised belief about your physique. As an instance, as soon as your belly produces a sound noise, you feel that means you're hungry. Or you are feeling nauseous and think you're sick. Both are examples of events that are noticed: you discovered a link once and decided to consider it. From the Rapid Weight Loss Diet," we're suggesting that you just turn that clinic around for this thought: "Think it, and you'll see it" It follows that you choose what to think, then your entire body works on it as authentic and which makes it real on your adventure.

Among the important messages, we expect that you will receive from the book is your mind-body hears that which you hear, what you say, all you presume, imagine, or picture in your head, and it can't tell the difference between what's actual and everything you envision.

Chapter 13:
All-natural Ways to Burn Fats

You do not need to invest thousands of dollars on the market's best fat heater to melt excess fats because you can burn fats naturally. Remember that this should be done with appropriate exercise along with a healthy and balanced diet if you want to discover how to burn tummy fat quickly for men. Keep in mind that you will certainly not have the ability to do this by focusing on a healthy diet or regular exercise alone. Another thing that you need to keep in mind is that losing stubborn belly fats could be impossible if you are to focus on a specific area alone. Right here are some techniques on how you can do it:

- **Reduce your caloric consumption:**

It is essential to consume reasonably and not as high as you want for you to eat fewer calories. The suggestion is that you should consume fewer calories than you shed. The lesser the number of calories you take, the much better. Perhaps replacing heavy meals with vegetables and fruits will certainly do the trick.

Counting calories is another essential action man need to take. Some men count calories, but they do not count the two to three beers they have in the evening, which is truly bad. Everything that goes right into your mouth needs to be noted.

- **Eating Healthy**

Learning how to burn belly fat quickly for men ought to include a healthy and balanced diet plan. Bear in mind that eating fast food, way too much coffee, and tea, soft drinks, and dealing with unneeded anxiety from school or work can only add up to your weight gain.

What you must find are the foods that can help you burn fats. Make sure you find out how to integrate healthy foods into your diet, and also, this ought to include foods such as vegetables and even fruits, lean meat, whole-grain grains, and beans, to name a few.

- **Eat foods rich in fiber.**

Fiber, as you know, is extremely useful in washing out contaminants, excess fats, and other unwanted bits in your body. You can eat a lot of vegetables and fruits day-to-day, and you can also consume alcohol lots of water. And if you can, get involved in the habit of drinking green tea. Green tea contains antioxidants and other compounds that help burn fats naturally.

- **Increase your physical activity:**

It is recommended to have three to five times weekly exercise regimen to lose weight. It should be that the exercise is at a moderate intensity to attain physical changes on your body. If you opt for a more vigorous aerobic activity, the better it is. When you don't have time to go to an aerobics class or enroll in a gym that is where the problem lies. To solve this, you just need to convert your everyday activities into a more active one. For example, replace your hobby of riding on an elevator with climbing on the stairs, walking to the office instead of riding on a car. There could be too much, and you just need to be creative on your exercise plan.

Fat loss for men is even more natural than it is for ladies. If a man just has a couple of pounds that they would like to lose, they can generally shed it rapidly. What might take a woman a couple of months to lose, a man can do it in a few weeks. Their bodies are just rigged in different ways, and they can do this, whether it's reasonable or otherwise. What are a few of the more crucial things you'll need to bear in mind to drop weight? One of the main formulae is exercise

Exercising regularly is an indispensable part of the process of weight-loss. Lifting weights is a great thing to obtain included within weight loss for men. They will, in turn, burn more calories when you train your muscle mass. They will be burning calories also while you're sleeping. This means that you will reduce weight quicker.

- **Limit Insulin Release**

Insulin is a storage hormone, and it can be lessened by removing unexpected dives in blood glucose. This is done only by eating more frequently. Primarily what you do is that you fuel your body much more equally throughout the day, and for that reason, your sugar degrees will be steadier. Snacks are essential and vital as they will help you to decrease blood insulin launch. In enhancement, you should drink more water, when feasible with lemon in it (or a few other citric juices).

- **Be positive and live a stress-free life.**

Sometimes, problems can add to your weight challenge. You will want to eat more if you get depressed. So, to avoid getting yourself into this situation, surround yourself with happy people in a healthy environment.

The Fat Burning Furnace

There are fat heaters available for men only, these unique formulas for men increase the testosterone level, thus boosting the fat loss process. They are specifically created to include many different active ingredients that are secure for men who prefer to reduce weight, melt fat, and improve muscle-building initiatives.

A common component in testosterone-based fat burners is high levels of caffeine.

L-Glutamine assists the muscles to recover after a man has completed his workout. Taken into consideration that reducing weight is a mixture of diet, exercise, and making use of fat burners having L-glutamine in this supplement improves its use because it also aids the immune system.

Lastly, cinnamon is contained in this fat burning supplement because it enhances the metabolic rate and diminishes the risks of diabetic issues.

A testosterone booster in the nutritional supplement of a man is always a great way to construct and melt the fat muscle mass too. L-Arginine is one more healthy protein item that expands the capillary, enabling more oxygen as well as nutrients to go into the bloodstream, inevitably enhancing the muscular tissues of a person.

You can choose from several fat burners for men available in the market; for instance, the ones pointed out over or any type of variety of combinations.

What about the ingredients type?

If not, do not take possibilities. Keep in mind any adverse effects related to the ingredients and take just the recommended dose.

Each of those items has various active ingredients and formulas. Nonetheless, some are better for men because they are targeted at not just the breakdown as well as the burning of the fat, but they are also aimed at bodybuilding. For your study, there are many organic food shops and even websites that specifically offer a selection of fat burners created for men.

Depending on the weight management requirements you want, and the current state of your health, your option of the fat burner needs not to be challenging to discover. But make sure that you include exercise in your strategy for weight reduction.

The truth is that men benefit nicely from programs like the Fat Burning Furnace. That's because as soon as they start, they begin to appreciate it. Before they understand it, the metabolic rate in their bodies has gotten much more energetic, and the weight simply starts to thaw off them permanently.

What happens is, as the people begin to do the regimens for twenty minutes a day and three days per week, they don't recognize that they have started to acquire a much leaner muscular tissue. And as that happens, the heating system is fueled, causing the fat to melt away simply.

You can prepare on shedding a great deal of body fat and get a lot of lean muscle mass. Not the big large muscles that men frequently link with the muscle contractors and body home builders.

While it may be helpful for you is you have a fitness center membership where you can use some professional equipment to help you along your journey, it is not a compulsory requirement but will produce the wanted results. A collection of dumbbells is one of the many things that will help you along your course to the goal and well worth the small investment if you don't already have some.

Similar to any routine that entails physical tasks, you must make sure that you are physically fit to do the procedures that will be needed. If you have a physical limitation that would prevent you from exercise or if you have particular troubles that need food policy, such as diabetes mellitus, you might want to get your doctor's approval before you begin.

If you want to learn how to burn belly fat fast for men, remember that this should be done with proper exercise along with a healthy diet.

Chapter 14:
The Four Golden Rules

Even however you may have instant success with the hypnotic gastric band, it's significant that you use the Four Golden Rules that are the foundation of my system. They help to support the progressions you are making. You may ask why you need the golden rules since you have a hypnotic gastric band; however, in certainty, those rules are at the core of all the healthy eating of all naturally slim individuals. Naturally, healthy individuals eat when they are hungry, they eat what they need, they focus on their food and appreciate it, and they quit eating when they are full.

As it were, healthy, thin individuals follow the Four Golden Rules naturally. It is a natural, healthy approach to eat. The splendid thing about your hypnotic gastric band is that it makes the physical changes that make it natural for you to follow the Golden Rules as well. How about we remind ourselves of them now.

Golden Rule One - WHEN YOU ARE HUNGRY, EAT!

When a few people hear me state this, they believe it's crazy. They say, "That is the issue, I can't quit eating, now, he's proposing that I eat." What I am saying is that when you are really physically hungry, get yourself a healthy meal, and eat. If you starve yourself, your body goes into "survival mode," and you slow your digestion. So, when you are genuinely hungry, and you eat, your body knows there will consistently be sufficient food, so it doesn't slow the digestion, and you have enough fuel in your "body's engine" to do the things you have to do. It's critical to make the distinction between genuine physical hunger and emotional craving. Real hunger starts gradually. It is clear and steady, and you feel it in your gut. It isn't activated by nervousness or by an emotional ache that goes ahead out of nowhere when you feel upset. It's anything but a response to fear, embarrassment, or outrage. It's anything but a plan to distract you when you are exhausted.

Real hunger is a straightforward physical feeling in your stomach. Sometimes, we confuse emotional distress for hunger. We suppose if we eat, we will feel much improved. Be that as it may, food doesn't fix emotions; it just covers them over incidentally. There are numerous, much better approaches to manage feelings than eating. If you speculate you need food because really you feel awful, you can use Havening to feel much better and afterward check in with your body and find whether you are actually physically hungry.

Recognizing Real Hunger

Proper physical appetite is a particular physical feeling, and with your hypnotic gastric band, you will think that it's simpler than at any other time to remember it. It will, likewise, be simpler to perceive when you are truly full. Be that as it may, for complete clearness and to ensure that you are precisely situated at both unconscious and conscious levels, I will request that you do a little psychological test that will help you in a split second and effectively perceive the signs for when you are really hungry and when you are full. If you have ever endured your way through a diet, you will have contorted your reaction to your body's natural signals. This activity will push your mind to recalibrate your stomach's natural sensitivity to craving and satiety.

1. Think about when you were super hungry—so hungry you felt swoon and even a crust of stale bread would have tasted delectable. Recall that.
2. Now, think about when you were totally stuffed—when you'd ate and eaten so much food that you were in pains, even nauseous. Remember that.
3. Do this a multiple time with the goal that you emphasize the contrast between being starving and stuffed
4. Alright, now unwind. Those two feelings are the extremes. You never need to feel both of those terrible emotions again. You never must be that hungry, and you never need to feel that full.

I have created a scale where one signifies being so hungry you are about to blackout and ten signifies being so full you believe you will explode. It will assist you with recognizing effectively where your body is whenever.

THE HUNGER SCALE

1. Physically blackout
2. Voracious
3. Genuinely hungry
4. Marginally hungry
5. Neutral
1. Six. Wonderfully satisfied

6. Full
7. Stuffed
8. Enlarged
9. Nauseous

Starting now and into the foreseeable future, NEVER go below three or over seven until kingdom thy come!

As you see, it gets simpler to live in the middle segment of the scale, your association with food, and your body will improve. You will feel more in charge, and like anything you practice for a couple of days, it will before long become natural. With your hypnotic gastric band, every one of these stages will be as clear as light. When you are somewhere in the range of 3 and 4, the time has come to eat. When you are somewhere in the range of Six and 7, the time has come to quit eating. With your hypnotic gastric band, you can't eat as much as in the past, so when you feel full, quit eating. Try not to attempt to eat more since it will sting to attempt to squash more food into your stomach.

Golden Rule Two - EAT WHAT YOU WANT, NOT WHAT YOU THINK YOU SHOULD.

When you make food prohibited, it turns into everything you can think about. That is the reason for your gastric band, and with my system, there are no illegal foods. It's game over. You wind up having it and beating yourself. That method for eating resembles battling with your body. It resembles driving a vehicle by stalling the accelerator and pulling on the hand brake. It is a misuse of fuel, and it trashes the vehicle. This disorder is intensified by dieting. Dieting mutilates your body's natural systems. All diets include constraining and denying the body. So, the body's reaction is to hunger for high-energy crisis foods to make up the deficiency as fast as could be expected under the circumstances. That is the reason individuals on diets all fantasy about high-fat, high-sugar foods like cakes and chips and French fries and frozen yogurt.

The more they diet, the more they need those foods. There is nothing amiss with any of them, coincidentally—but as you move away from dieting towards balanced nutrition, you might be shocked to see that what you need to eat starts to change. As you become progressively touchy, food that you never focused on begins to speak to you. You will likewise see that you start to support new food, in any event, when it sets aside more effort to cook or get ready. This happens because your body is never again attempting to save you from starvation. It isn't searching for a crisis energy fix. Presently it is allowed to move towards more noteworthy wellbeing. As you lose weight, it searches out the protein, nutrients, and minerals it needs to fix and explain your skin and fabricate your muscles.

The extraordinary thing pretty much every one of these progressions is you don't need to consider them by any stretch of the imagination. Your body's natural signaling system will control you. The more you focus on your body, the more you will understand that appetite isn't only a basic requirement for energy. You will start to see you are hungry for a particular food, for example, fish, or serving of mixed greens, or cake. You will see you lean toward one vegetable to another, etc. To summarize, dieters eat what a book discloses to them they ought to eat. Healthy individuals eat what their body truly needs.

Golden Rule Three- WHENEVER YOU EAT, DO IT CONSCIOUSLY.

This is potentially the most powerful suggestion I can give you, and what I am going to let you know is currently bolstered by various scientific research around the globe. When I state eat intentionally, I mean two things:

1. Focus on what you are eating, and that's it. Give your food your total attention. Concentrate on the food and NOTHING else!
2. Slow you're eating speed directly down. Slow down to about a fourth of your past speed and bite every mouthful multiple time. When individuals eat quickly, they flood their brains with happy chemicals (neurotransmitters), and they can't hear the signs from their stomach that say, "You are full." So, they end up crazy and gorging. It's significant that as you bite every mouthful of food, you put your blade and fork down and bite your food 20—yes, 20—times!

If you can't do this, I don't think I can support you, and I don't want to believe anybody can. It's a little favor you can do for yourself that comes with an enormous reward.

Concentrate on Your Food

You can eat anything you desire, at whatever point you need, so long as you give it your total, full concentration. That never implies, at any point, eat, and do something different simultaneously. When you eat, sit at a table, eat your food from a plate, using a blade and fork, and chew your food multiple times. This may appear to be a little ridiculous to you now. However, it is completely indispensable to retrain yourself to focus on each mouthful you are eating absolutely.

This will guarantee that you truly make the most of your food. Appreciate the taste and texture of your food, and truly notice it as you swallow it and feel how it fills your stomach. By focusing on eating, you will think that it's basic and simple to notice the satiety signal that you get from your hypnotic gastric band, and you will quit eating and be fulfilled sometime before you would have expected to because you will feel how rapidly your stomach tops off.

This is the one thing I need you to do to ensure you can encounter the advantage of your hypnotic gastric band and get more fit. Conscious eating is the manner by which individuals forget about their body's natural weight control system in any case. By eating deliberately, you regard your food, and you regard yourself. Research has demonstrated indisputably that individuals consistently eat more when they sit in front of the TV. Concentrate on your food solely. That implies no TV, but additionally no perusing while you eat. Try not to surf the Internet or answer messages or reply to your friends. Try not to drink liquor when you eat, because it dulls your attention and diverts you from the real food. Try not to snatch snacks while driving or tuning in to music or playing a game or using your telephone.

That may sound demanding; however, it is likewise incredibly useful since it implies that you should just ever eat food that you totally appreciate.

Chapter 15:
Tips and Tricks

To achieve your weight loss goals, you must be willing to let any fear and doubt you may have about hypnotherapy, go. It is not something that you can second guess, particularly not its effectivity and results-driven orientation. It is a solution used for many different reasons, even other than weight loss. Hypnotherapy for weight loss can help you overcome a negative relationship with food, one that may have formed over a period or throughout your entire life. It is something that can present you with proper results and that you can always be certain of.

Although it is not a diet or weight loss supplement, it fulfills a similar supporting role and serves as the foundation on the journey of living a more mindful lifestyle. Since the method thereof is focused on replacing old negative habits with new positive ones, it really helps one to overcome challenges faced when trying to lose weight.

Whether you want to opt for a one-on-one weight loss for hypnotherapy session or just listen to audiobooks online, both can serve you usefully.

Before you dive into the world of hypnotherapy, you should know that there's a lot more to it than you may have initially thought. Much like Yoga and meditation, in general, it serves a greater purpose as it leads you on to a mindful path of physical, mental, and emotional wellness.

Tips for hypnosis for weight loss

- Find the right hypnotherapist for weight loss for you. How would you go about doing this, you may ask? Instead of going the obvious route of searching for hypnotherapists online in your area, why not ask for recommendations instead? Honestly, what's better than asking a friend, family member, or acquaintance to recommend you a good hypnotherapist for weight loss? If no one you know, knows a hypnotherapist that is known for the outstanding jobs they perform, then you may want to check with your doctor and ask for advice. They should be able to recommend a qualified and results-oriented hypnotherapist for weight loss. To ensure you have the right hypnotherapist once you've found one, be sure to check with yourself whether their consultation felt as though it was thorough, whether the hypnotherapy program was adjusted to meet your needs if there were any, and whether the practitioner was helpful and answered all of your questions. When hypnotherapists allow for space between sessions, it's also an indication that you're dealing with a good hypnotherapist.

- Don't pay any attention to advertising. We live in 2019, which means that everything we see online is taken seriously. However, it shouldn't be. People are oblivious and susceptible to accept everything they read or hear, but when it comes to advertising, not everything can be trusted. Advertising should, ever so often, be disregarded and not taken too seriously as it can be very misleading. It's always better to conduct your own research before you simply accept that something is a certain way or not. In the case of hypnotherapy, since there are so many negative associations related to the practice, it's best to find out what's it all about yourself. As you can see from this useful set of information provided about hypnotherapy for weight loss, it is completely safe and probably nothing negative that you expected it to be.

- Get information about training, qualifications, and necessary experience. Before you pick a hypnotherapist, you must be sure about their basic information first. Do they run their own practice or operate independently? Are they certified and have a license? Ensuring that they also adhere to ethical standards, most preferably recommended by other medical physicians, you'll be assured that you are dealing with someone who knows what they are doing.

- Before choosing one hypnotherapist, talk to several first. Perhaps one of the best ways to find out whether a hypnotherapist is best suited for you is to talk with a few of them over a phone call first. This will take some effort, but it will be worth it in the end. You have to consider whether they can relate to you, care about your well-being and listen to your concerns, whether they are personable, accommodating, and professional. If they tick all the boxes, then you're good to go.

- Don't fall for any promises that may sound unrealistic. If a hypnotist tells you that their therapy session will help you lose weight fast, then don't even bother going to a single session. In reality, hypnosis for weight loss is a process that takes time. It can take anywhere between three weeks, up to three months to see your physical body change and to lose weight. Since your body and mind should first adjust, you need to allow time for it to do so. Hypnosis for weight loss isn't a fad, nor is it a means of losing weight overnight. It's also important to avoid hypnotherapists who suggest they will make you lose weight. Since they will only be talking during the session what they're telling you is not true whatsoever. What you can expect from a professional and authentic hypnotherapist, however, is a professional individual who takes responsibility for helping you to get where you want to go. This person should help you access your subconscious mind with ease, and help you bring it on board with a proper weight loss plan and possibly an exercise routine.

- Is your hypnotherapist of choice multi-skilled? Even though hypnosis is a terrific tool and can alter the mind's way of thinking about food, it goes hand-in-hand with nutrition. This is something you need to consider, especially whether your hypnotist has a good understanding of what it takes for you to lose weight sustainably and healthily. Many people focused on starting a weight loss journey don't necessarily know what they should do or what they should eat. When looking for a hypnotherapist, look for one that has a self-help coaching or some type of psychotherapy qualification, as well as a qualification/background in either nutrition or cognitive behavioral therapy.

- Find out the time you should engage in a program. This is quite important as hypnotherapy can become quite expensive if you're going to a professional for one-on-one sessions. If you prefer going to a professional rather than conducting the sessions at your home, you can choose to spread your sessions out over time to make it more affordable. Even though you may think that the sessions become less effective to achieve the overall effect, it works more effectively as your mind and body requires time to adjust. Time is also required as you change your old habits and replace them with new ones to lose weight.

- Ask your hypnotherapist if they can provide you with a program to maintain your progress at home. A recording particularly helps to allow you to spread out sessions over time. Listening to your weight loss hypnosis recording every day will keep you in check and help you stay motivated and focused.

- As your hypnotherapist if they can tailor-make your hypnotherapy weight loss program for you. If they agree to it, you can expect a weight loss hypnotherapy program that is much more effective than individualized hypnosis, offering treatments that may work better than ones that cater to everyone. Since every person is different compared to others, this makes a lot more sense. Sure, the general program will work, but a personalized one could offer you better results.

- Ask whether your program includes an introduction session. Starting with hypnotherapy for weight loss, you don't want to just dive right into it. It's important to take the necessary time, even if it's just an hour, to establish your needs and concerns regarding your current habits, lifestyle, and goals with your hypnotherapist. Ensuring that they care about your well-being and results instead of just taking you through the session is equally important. Taking the time to talk to your hypnotherapist and getting to know them better will help you feel more at ease and form a foundation of trust before starting with your hypnotherapy sessions.
- Establish the costs involved before starting with your sessions. Ensuring you know how much an initial consultation and each session costs will be another important factor you have to consider before choosing a hypnotherapist.

Lastly, you should view hypnotherapy as an investment in yourself and well-being, rather than an unnecessary expense. The context for this thought will realize once you engage in or completed your program.

Chapter 16:
Living a Healthy Habit Life

Get Yourself out of Solitary Confinement

In the United States, what do we do with the most exceedingly awful, most troublesome detainees? We put them in isolation. It's not unusual that isolation is a type of discipline since developmentally we are designed to look for association with different people. We should investigate the reasons why this is the situation. The initial three months after birth are regularly alluded to as the "fourth trimester," implying that babies should even now be in the belly. The explanation they don't remain there longer is that at around forty weeks (nine months) the human skull is still little enough to go through the birth trench. If we invest any more energy in the belly, our moms wouldn't have the option to bring forth us. So being conceived "too early" has been a vital exchange off in human advancement: we get the opportunity to have a vast, versatile cerebrum, yet we're conceived before we can make due all alone. Thus, people deal with their young for longer than practically some other vertebrate.

The connection is the explanation we feel mitigated and quiet within sight of protected and caring friends and family and bothered when we're isolated from them. Indeed, the sound of a crying infant rouses guardians to think about newborn children, to such an extent that tuning in to a crying infant is now and again utilized as a type of torment. Connection likewise clarifies why isolation (being isolated from different people) is a type of discipline. The impacts of connection don't cut off with the child-parent association, as we convey these forwards into our associations with mates and other notable individuals throughout our life.

Western culture is focused on the thoughts of independence and freedom. We get messages that we have to "love ourselves" and to have the option to "be all alone," and that it's useless to be reliant on others. The issue with these thoughts is that we're designed to work better when we have close, safe, and secure associations with others. At the point when we feel safely associated with others, we're better ready to investigate the world, handle difficulties, and be healthy. Indeed, the Western world is in the minority with its attention on independence. The majority of the world spotlights on cooperation, which organizes bunch cohesiveness and association. Collectivistic societies expect that intimate connections are essential for prosperity.

I prefer not to be separated from everyone else. I'm a social butterfly, and I feel uncomfortable when I'm without anyone else for extensive periods. In any case, since I comprehend human advancement better, I understand that my nervousness about being separated from everyone else is designed! It's not useless. There is parity. It may not be healthy to associate with individuals who are unsupportive or unpleasant just to abstain from being separated from everyone else.

So, for what reason am I discussing connections in a book about wellbeing practices? Studies show that intimate connections make us more beneficial. Individuals' injuries recuperate quicker on the off chance that they have secure, cozy connections, and they recoup from ailment quicker, have a more extended life, and are intellectually more beneficial. At the point when we're more youthful, having more individuals in our informal organization predicts better wellbeing, yet as we develop the nature of connections as opposed to the amount matters more. So, in case, you're perusing this reasoning, I don't have numerous old buddies, don't stress; having only one cozy relationship is sufficient for you to pick up these medical advantages. There's likewise proof of how healthy your companions are predicted how healthy you are. For instance, examines have demonstrated that if your informal organization incorporates many individuals living with heftiness, there is a more prominent possibility that you'll additionally be living with corpulence. There are various reasons why the healthy habits of our loved ones may impact our own, including hereditary qualities, for example, the affinity to gain weight or an inclination for sweet nourishments; living in comparable situations, for example, those with access to parks and strolling ways; and shared social standards, for example, having get-togethers that spin around food. Consequently, having an informal organization that centers on healthy habits can be critical to propping your healthy habits up.

No human is an island at any rate, the healthy ones aren't. Similarly, as you don't live alone in a vacuum, your healthy habits don't occur in a vacuum either. Individuals throughout your life can be the two partners and adversaries (typically accidentally) with regards to how you live, so your informal organization assumes a significant job in your capacity to participate in healthy habits and to carry on with a healthy and energetic life.

How to manage Other People...

At the point when I worked at the stoutness facility, I routinely heard stories from members about how they endeavored to keep snacks like potato chips or chocolate out of their home just to have a mate or youngsters or a parent bring them back in. "In what manner can I be healthy when my significant other continues bringing potato chips into the house!? I've asked him a hundred times to stop, he despite everything does it." Dealing with others is anything but a necessary errand. I could likely compose an entire book on this theme alone. Here are a couple of ways you can manage others in your life, every one of which I'll go over in more detail:

1) Change the things you can change.
2) Accept the things you can't change.
3) Do nothing.
4) Leave.

Change the Things You Can Change

If others in your interpersonal organization are not supporting your healthy habits, the initial step is to approach straightforwardly for their help. Emphatics is an expertise you can use to all the more likely impart your requirements and improve the probability that others in your life will bolster your healthy habits. There are loads of approaches to characterize confidence. I have thought that it was most straightforward to portray confidence (and the elective approaches to impart) in political terms:

1) Assertive correspondence resembles a big government: You get the chance to have your vote, yet your competitor doesn't generally win. You get the chance to express your needs; however, you don't generally get your direction.

2) Aggressive correspondence resembles fascism: you state what you require and consistently get your direction.

3) Passive correspondence implies you don't cast a ballot (or express a need), which frequently brings about your needs not being met.

4) Passive-forceful correspondence implies you don't express your needs yet ensure you get your direction. You don't cast a ballot (you don't express a need), yet you despite everything ensure you get the result you need. This correspondence style resembles utilizing secret activities to toss an upset and put your despot in power.

Self-assured correspondence includes plainly and legitimately communicating your emotions, assessments, and requirements while regarding the sentiments and privileges of others. It's about you expressing your requirements, not about whether they get met or not. How you act is inside your control; how the other individual reacts is outside of your control. The primary way you'll see whether individuals throughout your life can address your issues is if you approach explicitly for what you need. For instance, there's a distinction between saying, "I have to concentrate on my healthy habits, so I can't go to Ribfest with you," versus "I can't accept you're requesting that I go to Ribfest!" It's acceptable to remember that what you're asking of others may include a troublesome healthy habit for them as well. While rehearsing individual correspondence, it can assist with applying all the things you've found out about changing healthy habits up until this point. For instance, request a "do rather" objective as opposed to a "don't do" objective ("I'm attempting to eat more advantageous nowadays. Would we be able to go to a spot that has a plate of mixed greens bar rather than a spot that lone serves seared food?"). Or on the other hand, maybe you can utilize the 90 per cent rule: "At any rate once this week would we be able to eat at home as opposed to having inexpensive food?"

What disturbs everything? Changing your social style (the habits wherein you relate to other people) to be progressively sure is a significant task because common styles are discovered since at an early stage and for critical reasons. Since youths can't pick their family or their condition, they have to alter. Perhaps as a child, you made sense of how to put on a smile regardless, when you were upset, or you were a pleasing individual or found that yelling was the ideal approach to be heard. We all in all educated such modification procedures, and we can be thankful to our mind for comprehending ways for us to bear our childhood environmental factors, some of which were probably very irksome.

In any case, as adults, we have logically choice. We regularly get the chance to pick our assistants, our buddies, and our callings, so this procedure for perseverance may not now be flexible. It may not help you with being increasingly useful or continue with a genuine presence that issues to you. Sadly, when the mind finds a perseverance strategy that works, it needs to keep using it in any case. So, changing your social style in all probability clashes with an inside and out insightful and mainly practiced continuance method. Your voyagers may holler at you, and you may need to turn over many thunder strips and feel a full scope of the trouble. Luckily you presently have a full scope of aptitudes to manage these voyagers. (Just overview the last very few areas!) Remember, if you see passing on even more certainly as problematic, generously starting by being thoughtful with yourself. Exactly when you consider all that you consider yourself, your character, your character, your family, and your youthfulness, your correspondence style no doubt looks good. Prompt yourself that you didn't pick how your mind acclimated to past conditions, and you didn't pick your people or your immaturity. It's not your deficiency you're engaging in changing your correspondence style, yet it is your obligation, considering the way that no one else yet you can choose to change.

Chapter 17:
Discover the Satisfaction Factor

Components of Mindful Eating

A mindful meal can really enhance the joy and satisfaction you get from the meal. Rather than autopilot as you eat, you are attracted to a multi-sensory dining experience, such as vision, sound, taste, touch, smell, temperature, and texture. This will help you find the amount and type of food that can get the most satisfaction from your diet.

Gastrointestinal Taste

A hearty meal recognizes how perceptions of joy and taste change during the meal process. When you eat the first lump when you are hungry, it tastes like pure heaven, but can you take it at the end or leave it? This is called digestive taste disorders. If you are careful, this decrease in pleasure is a clue to know when you are going full.

Non-judgment

By approaching the dining experience with a sense of non-judgmental awareness, you can touch whether you are actually enjoying the dining experience and stop the voice of the inner food critic. Instead of saying "This cake is full of fat and chemicals", the positive, negative and neutral reactions to food are made with curiosity. "This cake is dry" or "This cake is fresh and delicious".

Cultivate Gratitude

Bringing mindfulness to the dining experience can also help to develop appreciation for the food we eat. That may mean we appreciate that there is something to eat at all.

Each year their magic purple and red foil eggs. Or you couldn't cook a meal from scratch due to a disability, and you could be hungry without it or eat potato chips for dinner, so a ready meal that was a perfect lifesaver in the case of.

It might be a farmer who raised your food. Or, after a long day at work, go to an eatery, which is open enough time to get bread and cheese on your way home. Appreciation for a safe food system means that you do not regularly suffer from food-borne illnesses.

Or for food technology that can keep milk in the refrigerator without the milk disappearing or froze in the hot moment. Perhaps the Uber Eats driver is riding a bicycle because he is working below the minimum wage and is difficult to bring back to you in the rain.

Even for a humble cheese toast or Heinz tomato soup, there are many reasons to appreciate the food we have to eat. Take a moment to thank it before you swoop down and eat it all lumpy. Mindfulness can be applied to almost every aspect of a dining experience, such as growing your own herbs and tomatoes, cutting vegetables, scooping ice cream, opening a pizza box for delivery, or a real dining experience. A mindful meal is a mindfulness that is particularly relevant to food and meal experiences.

So how do we do it?

People like to go really hard into this mindful eating thing, and while the enthusiasm is great, it doesn't always set you up for forming sustainable habits. My best advice would be to start small and build up from there.

The whole idea here is to work on minimizing distractions (phones, tablets, laptops, etc). A lot of us are living pretty frenetic lives, usually multitasking as we eat. Mindful eating is about lessening the distractions (when we can) and gathering information about the eating experience.

Let's break it down into steps.

Step 1 – Set an intention

Before you embark on mindful eating, it's helpful to check in with your intention for the practice; are you treating it like an experiment, with the aim of curiosity and intrigue as to what you might find?

Or are you coming at it as a way to control what you're eating and possibly eat less? It's important to be really real with yourself – are you coming at this as another diet? It's OK if that's where you're at, as long as you're being honest with yourself about it and not trying to trick yourself that it's something that it's not.

Then set an intention to come at this from a place of curiosity and non-judgement; you are simply bringing awareness to the eating experience and collecting information.

Step 2 – Start small

In terms of mindful eating, begin by focusing your attention on just one of these aspects of the eating experience. Notice if and when you get distracted, and gently bring your awareness back to that aspect of the food you were focused on.

Step 3 – One mindful meal

You are encouraged to set an achievable goal for your mindful-eating practice – maybe it's one mindful meal three times a week; maybe it's one mindful meal or snack a day.

It could even be just one mindful bite at the beginning of each meal. In fact, that's a pretty good place to start if you're new to mindful eating or a whole meal feels like too much. I try to aim for one mindful meal a day, usually lunch; where my focus is entirely on the meal I'm eating.

That doesn't mean I'm not bringing aspects of mindfulness to other meals, but this is the time I designate for really minimizing other distractions.

Step 4 – Be realistic

It's easy for mindful eating to become another thing to beat yourself up with if you don't nail it every time, but having the expectation that every single eating experience will be perfectly mindful and free from distraction is totally unrealistic for most people.

Some of you will have busy family lives, others will eat lunch with colleagues, and others will only manage a piece of toast in the car on the way to work. Think about ways you can gently apply aspects of mindfulness to these experiences, and if it doesn't always work out that way, that's OK too.

Step 5 – It doesn't have to be perfect

People have a tendency to want to perfect this mindful eating thing, but here's the thing: it doesn't have to be perfect. You're allowed to read a magazine or listen to a podcast. It's your call!! Gently incorporating mindfulness when you can is the key here. If you get lost in thought or distracted by your phone, no worries, just gently come back to the meal or snack when you notice your attention has wandered.

Step 6 – The elements of mindful eating

The components of meditation are to give you a sense of the elements of mindful eating you may want to place your attention on and to give you a sense of things you can think about.[1]

You don't have to use dead grapes; use whatever works for you to get a feel for mindful eating and use the outline opposite as a guide.

Chapter 18:
Motivational Affirmations

Motivational affirmations are phrases, sentences, or even words that will enable you to stay positive, be focused, and highly motivated. You need to choose these affirmations and use them on your daily basis. They are of great help as they will help you to meditate correctly on your weight loss. You can only reduce weight when you stay focused and positive. Being true to yourself and getting motivated every time will enable you to be able to control your weight. Even though these affirmations are numerous, you need to take a look at the ones I have detailed or illustrated the most common ones in the below paragraphs. It is good to note that, these affirmations, you can use them each morning after just waking up. They will sincerely help you to jump-start your day in a much higher note. It is a challenge thrown at you that you better try this and see how your life will drastically change. Your mindset will shift, and you will only be thinking positive. You will only be staying focused on your life, and this will increase your esteem within and outside your external world. Below are some of the examples that you need to go through with much keen.

You must embrace success. In every kind of situation or no matter the condition you are facing with, tell yourself about success. You need to talk about being successful every morning. The word "you can't" should not appear in your mind. Everyone has excuses. Some excuses emerge from fear of not trying. You need to stay focus and embrace the successful part of you. Don't get overwhelmed and overtaken by negative thinking about your success story. I challenge you to recite this affirmation every time you wake up. You will realize how important it is not only to your body but also in your external world. You need to feel unstoppable and fail to look at your excuses for not being successful. Negativity here is a BIG NO for you.

You must be calm always when faced with conflict. Conflicts are issues that always take you back to where you were. Conflict will automatically kill your daily morale leading to weak contributions of your abilities, especially within the organization and other sectors of life. You must try as quickly as possible to brush off annoyances easily. You must always agree with all sorts of disagreements so that the argument can end there. Tell yourself that you are more significant than what you are facing, and this should not drain you physically. Staying focused with a fit body and soul will make you lead a positive life.

At last, your weight will be highly controlled. You need to have that habit of doing this any time you are facing any conflict. It will only help you to stay positive and highly productive under your capacity. Reciting this affirmation every morning will be of great help. Try it as many as possible and help yourself to stay calm, relaxed, and comfortable.

You must choose to show love and gratitude every day. You need to know that life is always short, and concentrating on negativity is not good. It won't go well with you. It will only derail your success.

After all these, you must radiate elements of joy to yourself and have that love of your body. Showing all kinds of gratitude will enable you to lead a happy life. It will affect not only you but also the people around you. You must embrace this no matter what happens. Staying scorned and having negative thoughts only ages you as quickly as possible and leaves you with a body shape you never wanted. Be happy always, and show love to the surrounding. You must try this and believe me, and you will have a change within the next few weeks.

You must be impressive to others. Staying positive in life is an excellent deal to yourself. Use anything under your disposal to impress those who are around you. You need to be positive in everything to be as positive as you can and never underrate yourself. No one sent a letter to be born in a certain way, so you need to accept yourself the way you are. It will enable you to stay focus and lead a real-life every day. You need to develop this habit of saying this affirmation to yourself as it is of great help. It will also help you to start your day with big morale and a notch higher.

You are free to develop your reality. Realities are things that are with us no matter what happens. Therefore, you must strive hard to create your reality. No one is supposed to create you one since you are in a better position with much knowledge about yourself. You must have a choice and choose wisely in every kind of situation you might get yourself herein. Remember, nothing should stand in between you and your happiness peak. That apex of goodness should be your cup of joy, and no one should prevent you from creating this form of reality to you. Choosing your reality every day will make you stay positive and entirely focused on life. Besides, it will be of great help as far as your body is concerned. Remember to note that your life ultimately depends on the realities within you. You can lie to people around you, but believe me, and you cannot lie to yourself. Therefore, it will be of great advice that you keep this affirmation as it will help you live and stay positive. In the end, this will automatically reflect on your body shape and image.

You need to shed off any unimportant attachment. Unimportant attachments are things that no longer have any effect on your life. These are things that will only let you down, thus derailing your life goals of achieving a mind-set full of happiness. Your future success depends heavily on this, and for you to get at that position, you will need to detach yourself from anything that might let you down. You must note that anything might also mean any person. We have people in our lives that always try very hard to put us down. These types of people are afraid of your success in life. They will try their best to pull you down, no matter how hard you try to embrace only positivity in your life. It is time to get yourself going and void them like the plague. Remember, you must live and not only live but choose a pleasant experience. It will only be possible if you manage to refuse anything or anyone that is holding you back. Since I have said this, it is now my wish that you may practice this affirmation and use it as your routine daily. Practice makes perfect, and you will only realize that when you train.

You are enough just as you are. You must release that demonic notion of having comparisons between you and others. For you to stay specific, you must have some success standards. After developing all these, set your own goals and ambitions. Your vision should relate to your mission in life. After all these, you can now judge yourself using the basis of your success. Those rules and regulations you created in your success standards should enable you to judge yourself accordingly. Just know you are just enough the way you were born. You are a complete soul, and no part of you is lacking. So never try to make a comparison with others. You should note that affirmation helps in the realization of worthiness. Within a short period, you will be able to control your body image. Also, it will be of a great deal as it helps you in achieving some of the personal goals in life, and having a sound body is one of them.

You must be in a position to fulfill your purpose. The world should know your existence, and you must be ready to show your achievement. Showing your accomplished goals will need some positive deeds that lead to a successful life. On most occasions, people who trend are our trendsetters. They trend because of having done something positive or negative. They are then known all over the world. However, in this motivational affirmation, you need to focus on positive things. You need to be a trendsetter in showing the whole world what you are capable of offering. If you have been employed somewhere to sweep, you must clean until the country president cuts short his journey to congratulate you. Achieving your best is always one decisive way to be successful and lead a happy life free from stress and distress. Remember, this affirmation reminds you that no one has that power to stop you from doing or rather fulfilling your purpose in life. Sharing this thought every morning when you wake up will eventually get you somewhere. You must now stay focus and have this habit of telling yourself that no one can prevent you from achieving.

You must be results-oriented. In your daily life, you need to stay focus in life. Your primary focus should be on your results. It is through this that you will be able to realize your productivity.

To achieve this, you must be able to create some space for success. Get more success in your life. Avoid any derailing excuses that will only demean your reputation, thus lowering your success rate. Offer yourself these phrases every morning, and you will be in great joy for the rest of the day. You need not hold on excuses for failing to achieve something. Be yourself and have the ability to struggle until you reach that success in life. It is through this that your mind will have settled, giving you peace of mind. Peace of mind will enable you to lead a stress-free experience. It will reflect in your body image.

Be control of your won happiness. Happiness is an aspect of life that will initiate your feelings and moods towards a positive experience. It is like a gear geared towards your prosperous life. Staying positive here will be of great importance, and for you to realize this, you must take control of your happiness. Responsibility is a virtue, and being responsible will make you bold enough to face all kinds of situations. Your joy is your key to success, and no one should tamper with it. Make happiness your priority and be responsible for it. You must let no one make you angry. Angriness will only induce you with emotional feelings that will eventually affect your life more so your body image. Having seen this, you must now be in an excellent position to embrace this affirmation. Take it as an opener to your morning and employ it entirely in your life.

Chapter 19:
Gain Confidence

At this moment in time, there is nothing - nothing more important for you to do except to relax physically and mentally more and more. From this moment on, each and every breath will just help you to feel more relaxed. Each and every breath will help you to feel and to be calmer and calmer. And from this moment on, any sound outside this room will not affect or disturb you in any way. In fact, any sound outside this room will just help you to feel more relaxed. Any normal or outside noises will just help you to feel and just help you to be calmer and calmer.

Just listening now to the sound of my voice. The sound of my voice is just helping engage you into deeper relaxation. And in a few moments, I will count from ten down to one. With each and every number that I count from ten down to one, you'll you feel and just become more and more relaxed. With each and every number that I count from ten down to one, you'll just feel and you'll just become calmer and calmer. With each and every number that I count from ten down to one, you'll just drift deeper and deeper into relaxation. Not because I say so, but because it's the nature of the human mind to enjoy and to absolutely enjoy these wonderful levels of physical and mental relaxation. It really does feels good relaxing physically and it really does feel good just relaxing mentally more and more.

So, ten, beginning now to relax just more and more with every breath.

Nine, each breathe just helping you to feel more and more relaxed. Each and every breath just helping you to be calmer and calmer. Each breath is helping you to drift deeper and deeper...and relax...

Eight and all muscles in your body from the top of your head down to your muscles in your feet feel and become more relaxed now.

And seven, as the muscles in your body feel and become more and more relaxed; your mind becomes just calmer and calmer.

And six, your mind and your body continue to become more and more relaxed. Continue to become just calmer and calmer.

Five, drifting deeper and deeper relaxed. Just feeling and just becoming calmer and calmer.

And five drifts into four, and you drift deeper and deeper into relaxation.

Three, just enjoying this wonderful feeling, just enjoying this wonderful feeling of mental relaxation.

Two, calmer and more relaxed and becoming calm and just feeling more relaxed with each and every passing moment.

And one, and from this moment on, each and every breath you exhale just helps you to feel just helps you to be more relaxed. From this moment on, each and every breath just helps you to feel, and just helps you to be calmer and calmer. And from this moment on, with each and every day and hour that passes by you really are doing those things which you know inside your mind will bring success and will bring wealth into your life.

And one of the wonderful things about success, success is everywhere. You live and see that success. Success reveals itself everywhere you go. If you think about it, the computer that you're using is success. The pens that you write with are success. The car that you may drive is success. Success is revealed everywhere that you go. Each and every time you switch on a light that is success. And that success started with an idea, a wonderful idea that led to light being everywhere that you go, and ideas are powerful when they're acted upon. Ideas are almost like seeds and not acting on an idea it's just like having a seed in your hand. That seed in your hand is useless. That seed with that full potential to grow will not grow in your hand.

Just like an idea in your mind will not grow without action. That seed needs to be planted. That seed needs to be watered. That seed need action. And once the action is put into place that seed grows. That seed could begin to grow stronger and stronger and stronger just like an idea. An idea in your mind with action. That idea can simply grow and can become stronger and stronger and stronger. Life really is a wonderful fantastic journey. It's a wonderful journey where you can bring some wonderful things into your life. Life can give you what you want and as you receive life becomes a wonderful fantastic journey.

And every single day you're on this journey, every single day that passes by you get control you get to decide where this journey that you're on leads because one of the wonderful things about today is that all you can control is today. Today really is your past and future. And today is your future's past. So what things are you going to do today to bring success, to bring wealth into your life. Every single day you have decisions to make, choices to make. And those decisions, those choices that you make every single day will have an effect on your future. Today is really just your future's past. Just like today is your past's future. So what do you want your future to be? How do you want your future to pan out? What things do you want in your life? Just spend a few moments now thinking about those things.

Spend a few moments thinking what you want in your life. And I will give you a few moments as you think about those things now...

And as you think about those things, every part of you feels and just becomes more motivated now to bring those things into your life. As you think about those things, each and every part of you just feels and just becomes more and more determined to bring those things into your life. With every passing moment now, with every passing second of your life you really do believe more and more that you're going to bring those things into your life because in every single day now that passes by you're doing things and you're taking action. Turning those ideas into reality.

Success comes from doing - wealth comes from doing. You don't become successful; you don't become wealthy by just thinking about being successful by just thinking about being wealthy. Successful people become successful by doing things, by taking action. Wealthy people become wealthy by doing things and by taking action. And every single day, you're taking action. Every single day, you're making decisions and you're reaching your dreams. Every single day you're motivated, you're determined and you have a wonderful belief that you are going to bring those things into your life.

Each day, you're moving towards your goals. You're moving towards your dreams. You're moving towards wealth because every single day the decisions that you make move you towards where you want to be. Decisions and actions move you towards what you want or move you away from what you want. Isn't that how simple life can really be? A simple equation. Successful people in life are the doers. The successful people in life are people that take action. The successful people do more things, take more action than the people who only want to be successful.

Wealthy people take more action, make more decisions than people who don't have wealth in their lives. And with every single day now you're taking action, you can think of action, you can think of decisions of life being almost like a balance scale. And you can imagine on one side of the scale is success and wealth. The other side of the scale is being unsuccessful and even being poor.

With every single day that passes by, you have decisions to make whether to watch that TV program, deciding to stay in bed for another hour instead of doing something that you know would bring success into your life as putting weight to the side of being unsuccessful. Or by switching the TV off by getting out of bed and taking action. Doing something that you know will bring success into your life as putting weight onto that side of the scale of success; onto that side of wealth.

And with every single day now that passes you're using your time correctly. You're using your time wisely. Life really is one big clock that constantly is ticking by, you cannot speed time up. You cannot slow time down. It's constantly ticking by. Tick tock. Tick tock. And things that you do each day will predetermine what will future will be. One of the wonderful things about time is everybody has the same amount of time.

Every single day starts the same amount of time. Every day you have 24hours to use. You have 1,440 minutes to use. And you have 86,400 seconds every single day. And every single day, things that you do with that time is either putting weight on that side of success and wealth or putting weight on that side of unsuccessfulness, being poor and every day you really are now making the right decisions. You're making the right decisions. You're putting that weight towards success. You're putting that weight on the side of wealth. And wealth and success because of that is really coming into your life. You really are on a wonderful fantastic journey.

It's also important to realize on this journey, you will do things and you will fail. You may try something and it might not go correctly. And in a way that could be life testing you, seeing how much you really want this. If you do something and fail and quit, then you didn't want it bad enough. Many of the inventions if not all of the inventions we see around us came about by many mistakes by many so called famous. Thomas Edison, a report of one says how it felt to fail 9,999 times to which Mr. Edison replied "I never failed once. I found 9,999 things which didn't work. And for those 9,999 things which didn't work, I found one thing that did work by doing something and realizing what didn't work.

You can change the approach. You can do something differently. It was all part of that wonderful journey and being on that wonderful journey brought that invention to success. That invention that's all around us each time you switch on a light. That light was first just an idea. An idea in someone's mind. And that wonderful idea is now everywhere because of action. Because of the decision of using time correctly.

Chapter 20:
Fall in Love with Your Body

Stop waiting for the perfect occasion to be at ease with your body and start enjoying it from today. Because the best time to love yourself is now.

Weight loss is considered a battle for a reason. It is usually normal that, when you try to lose weight, you often feel as if you are in a war against your body. This is why it is important that you are committed to the effort you are making so that you do not self-sabotage.

This does not mean that you should feel that your body is your enemy for not having certain measures. In fact, when you have such negative thoughts, they may play against you and it will be much harder to achieve your final goal.

Fall in love with your body

- **Did you see for now?**

For starters, clothes are very influential and show how you perceive yourself. It is not about buying clothes for the best brands, but the best size according to your body.

It may happen that you want to cling to clothes that you may not have left in the hope that "one day it will be worth it." Or maybe you refuse to buy nice new clothes because you're waiting to reach your desired weight to do so.

In both situations, your closet is belittling the body you have at that time. To really love your body, you have to be aware of the way you look with your current weight.

It is not bad that you invest in some articles of clothing that help you see and feel good. When you don't know what to choose, it's time to explore new options. Therefore, allow yourself to see what kind of garment and colors are best suited to your body and accentuate your positive features.

- **Consent your body before sleep**

It's good that you have a routine that allows you to take care of yourself and feel good. You can get a manicure, pedicure or facial treatments that allow you to feel better about how you look at bedtime.

It is also a good idea to resort to spa therapies, such as relaxation massages, from which you can also obtain benefits for weight loss. While it is true that not everyone has the money for frequent visits to the spa, this does not prevent you from having your own spa nights at home.

It can be as simple as buying some low-cost ingredients that allow you to feel pampered. For example, moisturizers and Epsom salt baths help relieve tired muscles and renew energy. You can also buy fresh and sexy nail polishes.

- **Take a photo session**

If you have already tried the first suggestions and you are still not in love with your body, we recommend that you do a photo shoot for yourself. It may sound like a slightly silly option, but it isn't.

Many photographers do sessions for people who are not models. And by the hand of a team of experts, they can make you look and feel like one of them. In addition, it is difficult for you not to love your body after seeing such a splendid image of you.

- **Why don't you like your body?**

Take the time to analyze if you are really dissatisfied with your body or if you are simply being carried away by the opinions of others. There is a possibility that what those around you think is influencing you.

In many cases you may worry too much about other people's opinions when in reality you feel comfortable with who you are. Who has control over your body are you? And, if you want to change something in it, it must be because you consider what you really want and not what others want.

- **There is no ideal body**

Not even in the fashion industry. With each new trend, specialists must choose what type of body will look best with their designs. In real life the thing is very different.

If everyone chose to have a "standard" body, life would be very boring. We are all different, from the shape of our bodies to our tastes. There is no ideal prototype of a perfect body that everyone likes. It is important that you appreciate yourself as you are, an individual being and very valuable for being unique.

- **You are not forbidden to do things**

Many times, to feel self-conscious it will be difficult for you to leave your comfort zone. However, if you just do not do activities like going to the pool with your friends for feeling ashamed when wearing a swimsuit, you will be missing out on wonderful moments in life that you may not be able to recover.

Do not let feelings against your body prevent you from enjoying. If you let yourself be dominated by sadness, hate or perhaps contempt for yourself, you will feel worse and worse and it will be harder for you to value the little things in life.

- **Allow yourself to be happier with who you are**

To despise your body and complain does not solve the problems in any case. If there really is something you want to change, strive, act and fight to achieve it.

Respect yourself for being who you are, and you will see how everything will begin to flow more positively in your life. No matter what method you use: take your time to take care of yourself and be grateful for the fortune of being yourself.

Chapter 21:
Positive Impacts of Affirmations

You control the fundamental fixings that make self-hypnosis work for you. These are similar fixings that make your experience of achievement for any objective you pick. Let us take a gander at every component and how you may utilize it to perform for you.

Motivation

Motivation is the vitality of your craving, of what you need. Needing is an inclination that you can control. For the greater part of your life, you have chiefly controlled your craving or needing by restricting it or denying it. You might be truly adept at controlling your wants and needing in certain regions and powerless or natural in others. Since this is a "diet" book, you may have just set yourself up to hear that this "diet" will resemble the others that have mentioned to you what you should deny yourself or breaking point. That is, different diets have mentioned to you what not to need, and the accentuation may have been about "not needing" a few nourishments that you have developed to cherish. Welcome to another method of treating yourself; we will urge you to show signs of improvement at "needing." Denial is excluded from Rapid Weight Loss Hypnosis.

Your motivation is a key factor, one of the fundamental fixings. We need you to center your vitality of needing not toward food yet toward the motivation that unmistakably tells your mind-body what you need it to make: flawless weight. We urge you to get great at needing your ideal weight. Here is a model. Let us state that you are in a pool, and out of nowhere, you take in a significant piece of water. At that time, you need just a single thing, a breath of air. It feels like decisive, and a breath of air is the main thing on your mind as of now. The needing is so serious and powerful that it dominates every single other idea and urges you to take the necessary steps to get that breath of air. That is the amount we need you to need the weight and self-perception that you want.

Conviction and Believing

Convictions are those musings and thoughts that are valid for you. They don't need to be deductively demonstrated for you to realize that they generally will be valid for you. Insite that, you know about it or not, your activities, both mindful and subconscious, depend on your convictions. Even though your convictions are as contemplations and thoughts, they shape your experience by influencing your activities throughout everyday life. If you accept that creatures make great sidekicks, you most likely have a feline or canine or parrot or a ferret or two. If you accept that espresso keeps you alert around evening time, you likely don't drink espresso before hitting the sack. The power of accepting lets you impact your body in manners that may appear to be bewildering. Fake treatment reactions, where people react to an inactive substance as though it were genuine medicine, are regular instances of how convictions are knowledgeable about the body. If an individual truly accepts that he will get well when taking specific medicine, it will happen whether the tablet contains a prescription or is inactive. Similarly, if an individual truly accepts that he can accomplish high evaluations in school, it will occur. If an individual truly accepts that he can achieve his ideal weight, it will occur.

Recollect your pretend games as a kid. Your capacity to imagine is similarly as solid now as when you were exceptionally youthful. It might be somewhat corroded, and you may require a touch of training, yet when you permit yourself to imagine and let yourself have faith in what you are imagining, you will find a powerful apparatus. You will find this is a brilliantly viable approach to convey your goals, those messages of what you need, to the entirety of the phones and tissues and organs of your body, which react by bringing that goal into reality for you. We can't state this enough: musings are things. The musings, the photos, the thoughts you put in your mind become the messages your self-hypnosis passes on to your mind-body, eventually transforming your ideal body into reality and imagining is picking what to accept and getting retained in those thoughts. Similarly, as an amplifying glass can center beams of daylight, you can center your psychological vitality to make your considerations, thoughts, and convictions genuine for your body.

Desire

You may not generally get what you need, yet you do get what you anticipate. Desires contain the vitality of convictions and become the aftereffects of what is accepted. Here is a case of how to "anticipate." When you plunked to peruse this book, you didn't analyze the seat or couch to test its capacity to hold your weight. You just plunked without contemplating it. You didn't need to consider it, because a piece of you is sure, and has such a great amount of confidence in the seat, that you simply "anticipated" it to hold you. That is the way to expect the ideal body weight you want. Remembering this, be mindful of what you state to yourself as well as other people concerning your body weight desires. "I generally put on weight over the special seasons."

Mind-Body in Focus

Every one of the fundamental fixings can create powerful outcomes when centered inside the mind-body. Nonetheless, when these fixings are adjusted appropriately inside the procedure of self-hypnosis, their viability has amplified a hundredfold. Self-hypnosis is a procedure for creating your world. You may think this sounds mystical or unrealistic. However, that is comparative with what you have encountered as yet in your life. These thoughts might be exceptionally new to you. Here is a case of the "relative" idea of new thoughts. Envision that you are given a personal jet that is flawlessly equipped with sumptuous arrangements and a very much prepared team. It is a brilliant blessing, and you get the opportunity to show this designing wonder to certain people who have seen nothing like it.

Your subconscious (mind-body) utilizes the mix of what you need (motivation), what you accept, and what you expect as a plan for activity. The outcomes are accomplished by your mind-body (subconscious), and not by deduction or breaking down. If an individual contact a virus surface that she accepts is hot, she can create a rankle or consume reaction. Then again, an individual contacting an extremely hot surface reasoning that it is cool may not deliver a consume reaction. Individuals who stroll over hot coals while envisioning that they are cool may encounter a warm physical issue (some minor singing on the bottoms of their feet). Yet, their invulnerable framework doesn't react with a consume (rankling, torment, and so on.) because their minds advise their bodies how to respond. Once more, it is the arrangement of every one of the three of the basic fixings that make this conceivable:

- •wanting to do it
- •believing it conceivable
- •expecting to be fruitful

This is the way to progress. Your body completes your convictions. Your convictions direct your activities, which like this, shape your experience.

Some portray this procedure as creating your prosperity or creating your involvement with life. In our way of life, we see this depicted inside the motivational and positive mental disposition writing. It very well may be seen in numerous zones of mysticism. You can likewise think back to the people of yore and see it depicted in the provisions of the authentic period. An individual a lot smarter than we are stated, "It will be done unto you as per your conviction." In the current period of integrative medication and brain research, we call it self-hypnosis or mind-body medication. There are currently various logical examinations that exhibit astonishing outcomes for torment control, wound mending, physical modification, and a lot of more medical advantages than we recently suspected conceivable.

Picking Your Beliefs

You can pick your convictions. You may decide to accept what you see, in the feeling of "See it to trust it" or "Truth can be stranger than fiction." This is simple to do. You experience something with your faculties, and that is a natural method of picking whether it is reasonable or not. However, you may likewise decide to trust it first and afterward observe it, which may require some training. The vast majority think that it's simpler to let the world mention to them what is valid or what to accept. The TV, media, papers, books, instructors, and specialists besiege us with what to accept. You grew up finding out about the world and yourself from numerous outside sources. This prompted a recognizable example of watching and accepting data about the world from outside yourself, and you picked which data to make a piece of your conviction framework. This included convictions about your body. For instance, when your stomach makes a thundering sound, you accept that it implies you are ravenous. Or then again, you feel queasy and trust you are wiped out. Both of these are instances of watched occasions: you watched an association once and decided to trust it.

In Rapid Weight Loss Hypnosis, we are suggesting that you turn that training around with this thought: "Trust it, and you will see it." This implies you initially pick what to accept, and afterward, your body follows up on it as evidence and makes it genuine, you would say. One of the significant messages we trust you will get from this book is that your mind-body hears all that you hear, all that you state, all that you think, picture, or envision in your mind, and it can't differentiate between what is genuine and what you envision. It follows up on what you need, accepts, and anticipate. In light of this, which of these announcements would assist you with encountering the ideal weight you want: "I simply take a gander at food and put on weight" or "I can eat anything, and my weight remains the equivalent"? The last mentioned. In any case, which articulation do you by and by accept to be valid for you? Once more, it will be done unto you as indicated by your conviction. We will assist you with the thoughts, language, and pictures that plan compelling hypnotic proposals, yet you have all-out command over what you decide to accept.

As you read the thoughts of this book and hear the hypnotic recommendations offered during the trancework on the sound, you will settle on numerous decisions for yourself. We wholeheartedly urge you to decide to trust it so you will see it for yourself. Your subconscious (mind-body) can't differentiate and will follow up on what you select in any case. Why not select what you truly need?

The Energy of Emotions

Not all considerations and convictions show themselves into your experience. Just those that have the vitality of your sentiments (feelings), alongside your conviction and your desire that something will occur, will show themselves. Your sentiments or feelings are a type of vitality that impacts this procedure of creation.

Chapter 22:
Tips to Help You Succeed with No Stress

For the most part, when we are talking about losing weight and making sure that we can get our health in the right order that we would like, we are going to focus just on the exercise and the diet. Both of these are important. One is going to ensure that we are able to lose weight and keep our hearts as strong as possible in the process and is known for helping to fight off a lot of the different diseases that are out there. But the other one will help to reduce weight and can ensure the body is getting the nutrients that it really needs as well.

However, there are a few other options that we are able to do that can make it easier to lose the weight and eat fewer calories overall, so that we can lose the weight without all of the stress. These are going to be so effective when it comes to reducing your own weight and can prevent some of the weight gains that we are worried about seeing in the future. Some of these are going to include:

Slow Down and Chew

We have to start slowing down when it is time to eat our meals. We need to give the brain some time to process what you are eating and to know when you have had enough to eat. When you chew the food all the way through, it is going to force you to slow down in your eating, and it is going to be associated back with a decreased amount of food that you take in. It can make you feel full faster and you will take on smaller portion sizes.

How fast you are able to finish your meals can also have a big effect on your current weight. And fast eaters in these studies were also the ones who are more likely to be obese.

This is an easy thing to fix. You can set a timer and not allow yourself to eat faster than that at any time. You can also make it be set up so that you count how many times that you chew each bite, and then take a drink of water in between. This is going to be an easy way to help you to slow down and will make it easier to eat less at the meal.

Go with Smaller Plates

You will find that the typical food plate is a lot bigger than it used to be. This is a trend that is going to contribute to weight gain because using a smaller plate can help you to eat less as your portions are going to look a lot larger than they are. This is a good way to ensure that you are going to trick your mind about how much it is eating.

On the other hand, when you work with a plate that is a lot bigger, it is going to make a serving, even one that is bigger, look smaller. You will be more likely to add on more food and eat more than you should. This means that you can use this to your advantage. If you are going to eat a lot of healthy foods, go with the bigger plate, so you take on bigger portions of it and get more of that good stuff.

But if you are going to eat foods that are not as healthy, then go ahead and go with the plates that are smaller.

Add in the Protein

Protein is going to have some powerful effects on appetite. It is able to help us increase our feelings of fullness, can help us to reduce your hunger, and will make it easier to eat fewer calories. This may be because protein is going to affect several hormones that play a role in hunger and fullness, including the ghrelin hormone.

There is one study that found when we increase our protein intake from 15 percent to 30 percent of our calories, it made it easier for participants to take in 441 fewer calories per day and then lose 11 pounds over a 12 week period on average, and this was all without intentionally restricting any of the other foods that the participants were eating.

A good way to use this is with your own meals. If you are eating a breakfast that is full of grains, for example, then switching to a meal that is higher in protein may be a good place to start. In one study, it found that obese and overweight women who had eggs as part of their breakfast were able to eat fewer calories at lunch compared to those women who at a breakfast that was based more on grains.

Eat the Fiber

Eating foods that are rich in fiber is another way for us to make sure that we increase our satiety, which is going to help us to feel fuller for a longer period of time. Studies are also showing us that one type of fiber, which is known as viscous fiber, is going to be really helpful when it comes to weight loss. This one is so good because it is able to increase the amount of fullness that we have, and it is able to reduce the foods that we intake.

Viscous fiber is going to form a gel when it comes in contact with water. This gel is going to increase some of the nutrient absorption time and it is going to slow down how the stomach is able to empty out as well. viscous fiber is something that we are able to find in foods that are planted, so we are going to find it in places like flax seeds, oranges, asparagus, Brussels sprouts, oat cereals, and beans as well. Here is also a weight loss supplement out right now that is known as glucomannan and it is going to have a high amount of this viscous fiber as well.

Drink Water Often

We also have to make sure that we are drinking enough water on a regular basis because this will help us to fill up our stomachs so that we eat less and lose weight in the process. This is going to happen even more when we make sure to drink before a meal. There was one study in adults that found that drinking about 17 ounces of water about half an hour before a meal would help to reduce the amount of hunger that was felt and could help to lessen how many calories the individual was going to take in.

Those participants in this study who took the time to drink more water before their meals were able to lose 44 percent more weight over a period of three months compared to those who did not have the water before their meals. If you are able to replace some of the regular drinks that you like to have, which are loaded with calories, such as juice or soda, with water, it is possible that the weight loss that you are experiencing will be even higher.

Keep the Portions Small

In addition to those bigger plates that we were talking about before, you will find that portion sizes have really seen an increase over the past few decades, especially when we go out to eat. These larger portions are going to encourage people to eat more and can be linked back to an increase in weight and obesity overall as well.

In fact, there was one study in adults that fond that when the appetizer with the dinner was doubled, it was able to increase the number of calories that were taken in by 30 percent. You will find that serving yourself just a little bit less could be enough to help you to eat fewer calories, and if it very unlikely that you would even notice the difference.

Don't Eat Neat the TV

Paying more attention to what you are eating could help you to take in fewer calories overall. Those who eat while they are on the computer or watching a show could easily lose track of the amount they are eating.

In addition, being absent-minded when it came to the meal would have a bigger influence on how much you took in later in the day. Those who were more distracted during a meal would eat 25 percent more calories at later meals than those who paid more attention. If you are in the habit of consuming meals while watching TV or using some kind of electronic device, then it is likely you are eating more without noticing. These are calories that will add up and can have a big impact on your weight over time.

Try to Avoid Stress and Sleep More

Now, if you are a parent, you probably read the thing above and started laughing. Sleeping well and avoiding all of the stress can seem almost impossible when you are a parent, and you have a bunch of things to keep track of for your children. And if your children are not sleeping through the night yet, getting that sleep that you need may seem almost impossible as well. This is also why a lot of parents are going to gain weight when taking care of their children and it is a good example of why we need to pay a bit more attention to our own sleeping styles to ensure that we get enough.

When it comes to your health, people are often going to neglect taking care of their stress or getting enough sleep. Both of these are going to have really powerful effects on your weight and your sleep. A lack of sleep is going to be enough to disrupt the hormones that are meant to regulate the appetite, the hormones of ghrelin, and leptin. Another hormone, known as cortisol, is going to get elevated any time that you are feeling stressed out.

Having these hormones fluctuate on a regular basis is going to increase your hunger and your cravings for foods that are not all that healthy, which is going to lead us to take in more calories in the process. In addition, studies have shown how a chronic level of sleep deprivation and chronic levels of stress especially when the two are combined, could be enough to increase your risk of several diseases, including obesity and type 2 diabetes.

Chapter 23:
Enjoy the Experience of Nurturing and Taking Care of Your Body

Progressing in the direction of Goals

Individuals in recuperation offer the accompanying recommendations:

- Concentrate on your qualities.
- Concentrate on tackling issues.
- Concentrate on the future as opposed to exploring harms from an earlier time.
- Concentrate on your life rather than your disease.

As you take a shot at your recuperation, you should record a portion of your principle objectives. These objectives can be present moment and effectively attainable, or you can begin recognizing greater, all the more long-haul objectives that you need to work your way towards. It's useful to consider little strides to take toward them over a specific measure of time, similar to a week or a month. Make sure to praise yourself for any triumphs. Accomplishing objectives - even little ones - is an indication of expectation and achievement.

Creating objectives for recuperation can be precarious, particularly on the off chance that you aren't sure what it is that you need to achieve. Think about your inclinations, things that bring you delight and things that keep you roused. Likewise, consider the things you need, similar to where you need your life to go or what you would accomplish a greater amount of if you could. Having a profound interest in the objectives that you set will expand the odds of finishing them.

When you have defined objectives for yourself, you have to make sense of what things are important to achieve those objectives. Be clear concerning why you set this goal and how your life will be diverse once this objective is accomplished. You ought to likewise consider the qualities and aptitudes that you have that will assist you with accomplishing your objective. Attempt to include important, emotionally supportive networks and assets that can help you through the procedure if and when you need it. At long last, make sure to remain concentrated on the objective and not on the challenges you may be having. Keep a receptive outlook, and realize that you may hit hindrances en route. Recuperation is no simple errand, and concentrating on the negative encounters will make things harder.

Make a diary or scrapbook with pictures and clippings to help keep up your objectives. Keeping a diary or scrapbook is a good method to follow your objectives and help you to remember the things you've achieved and the things you despite everything intend to achieve. Keep on including new astonishingly up. Recuperation is a consistent procedure and proceeding to set objectives for yourself will keep you inspired to reach and look after health.

Care for Yourself

Taking great consideration of yourself is foremost to the achievement of your recuperation procedure. Individuals in recuperation find that their physical, profound, and enthusiastic wellbeing are altogether associated and that supporting one bolsters the others. Dealing with all parts of you will improve the probability that you remain well.

To help bolster you in your recuperation, you can get to a three-minute screening apparatus and progress screen for wretchedness, uneasiness, bipolar disorder, and PTSD. Snap here to take the screener or imprint your advancement.

A few tips for self-care include:

- Live healthily, eat well nourishments, get enough rest, practice consistently, and keep away from medications and liquor. Oversee pressure and go for ordinary restorative registration.
- Practice great cleanliness. Great cleanliness is significant for social, medicinal, and mental reasons in that it decreases the danger of disease. However, it additionally improves how others see you and how you see yourself.
- See companions assemble your feeling of having a place. Consider joining a care group to make new companions.
- Attempt to accomplish something you appreciate each day. That may mean moving, viewing a most loved TV appear, working in the nursery, painting or perusing.

- Discover approaches to unwind, similar to contemplation, yoga, getting a back rub, washing up or strolling in the forested areas.

Reinforce Your Connections

The significance of consolidating satisfaction, soul, and unwinding in your life has numerous ramifications in creating flexibility (the capacity to recoup from a sickness) and remaining solid. The four C's to bliss, soul, and unwinding are: associate with yourself, interface with others, associate with your locale, and make happiness and fulfilment.

Associate with Yourself

Significantly, you check in with yourself occasionally. If you don't, at that point, you may not understand that things are changing or gaining out of power. Checking in with yourself permits you the chance to assess where you are in your recuperation. You may find that you have to straighten out what venture of your activity plan you are on or attempt diverse adapting tools.

If you have had low occasions in the past, you see how hard it tends to be to escape those spots. Realizing all that you can about your emotional wellness condition will help let you realize that your tough occasions are not your issue. Making a rundown of achievements that you have accomplished is a decent asset to turn around to when you are feeling low.

Another tool that may help you is to diary about your encounters. Keeping a diary is an extraordinary method to find out about yourself. Being legit in your diary is significant; in your diary, you should don't hesitate to allow your gatekeeper to down. That will assist you in finding how you truly feel and vent your worry in a non-undermining way.

Another strategy for interfacing with yourself is to turn into a promoter and offer your story. There has been a great deal of research that investigates the intensity of narrating as a type of treatment. Sharing your encounters through composition or talking is a significant phase of recuperation. Similarly, as you are bolstered by perusing the musings and encounters of others, you can likewise be the individual that helps lift another.

Interface with Others

Investing energy with constructive, cherishing individuals you care about, and trust can ease the pressure, help your disposition and improve how you feel in general. They might be relatives, dear companions, individuals from a care group or a friend advisor at the nearby drop-in focus. Numerous people group even have warmlines (free hotlines run by individuals with psychological wellness conditions) that you can call to converse with somebody and get peer support.

Research focuses on the advantages of social association:

- Expanded joy. In one convincing investigation, a key distinction between exceptionally glad individuals and less cheerful individuals was acceptable connections.

- Better wellbeing. Dejection was related to a greater danger of hypertension in an ongoing investigation of more seasoned individuals.
- A more drawn out life. Individuals with solid social and network ties were a few times less inclined to kick the bucket during a 9-year study.
- Association happens when you get:
- Solid assistance, for example, having a companion get your children from school;
- Passionate help, such as hearing somebody state, "I'm extremely sorry you're having such an intense time";
- Viewpoint, such as being reminded that even the moodiest young people grow up;
- Exhortation, for example, a proposal to design a week after week date with your life partner;
- Approval, such as discovering that different people love perusing train plans as well.

Do you have enough help? Inquire as to whether you have at any rate a couple of companions or relatives who:

- You feel good to be with;
- Give you a feeling that you could disclose to them anything;
- Can assist you with taking care of issues;
- Cause you to feel esteemed;
- Pay attention to your interests.

Interface with Your Community

An incredible method to feel sincerely solid and strong amid stress is to feel associated with a wide network. Consider the things you like to do. You can grow your interpersonal organization by investigating a network association that unites individuals who share similar premiums. For example, numerous networks have nearby biking, climbing, or strolling gatherings. Is there something you've for a long while been itching to do like gain proficiency with another dialect? Take a class or join a nearby gathering. You additionally may discover the help you need through neighborhood support bunches for a particular issue like child-rearing, managing a medical issue, or thinking about a friend or family member who's evil.

Or then again consider volunteering with a network association that helps fill a need. Here are a few hints to ensure your volunteer experience works for you and doesn't turn into an extra wellspring of stress:

- Get the correct match. Consider what sort of work you like to do, in light of your inclinations, aptitudes and accessibility. Think about making this a rundown for simpler comprehensibility. Do you like to peruse, compose, manufacture things, fix things, or sort and arrange? Do you have an extraordinary field of information that you could educate to battling understudies as a guide or mentor? Is it accurate to say that you are particularly worried about vagrancy or contamination? Do you love to garden or work in an office? Do you communicate in another dialect? Do you should be at home, and carry your humanitarian effort home with you? Whatever your circumstance and your inclinations, there is most likely a volunteer chance to make an incredible commitment in your locale. Volunteering will assist you with building solid associations with others - a demonstrated method to secure your psychological well-being.

- Make the most of it. You need your volunteer time to have any effect, so pose inquiries to ensure the association utilizes volunteers proficiently and beneficially. Ask what volunteers do, where and when they do it, and whether a representative is accessible with data and direction when required.

Make Joy and Satisfaction

Living with a psychological wellness condition can be exhausting inwardly, genuinely, and intellectually. Specialists have discovered that nice sentiments can help your capacity to manage pressure, tackle issues, think deftly, and even fight ailment. Dealing with your body inwardly, truly, and intellectually through making euphoria and fulfilment is a significant piece of living with or without an emotional well-being condition.

Studies show that:

- Snickering diminishes torment, may support your heart and lungs, advances muscle unwinding, and can lessen nervousness.

- Positive feelings can diminish pressure hormones and construct enthusiastic quality.
- Relaxation exercises offer an interruption from issues, a feeling of ability and numerous different advantages. For instance, in one investigation watching twins, the person who partook in recreation exercises was more averse to build up Alzheimer's disease or dementia than their twin.

A few hints to appreciate life and unwind:

- Accomplish something you wanted to do as a child. Go through the sprinklers, dangle from the playground equipment, or make a wreck with finger paints.
- Accomplish something you've for the longest time been itching to do. In case you don't know how to take a class or search for a neighborhood bunch devoted to the action.
- Watch or tune in to parody. Through video, digital broadcast, or site. Or on the other hand, get a giggle as it was done in the old-fashioned days - through the funnies segment.
- A remedial back rub. A back rub can mitigate muscle strain, animate the body's regular painkillers and lift your resistant framework. It can likewise assist you with feeling not so much restless but rather looser.

Chapter 24:
Eat Healthy and Sleep Better with Hypnosis

Make yourself comfortable.

Find the perfect sleep position.

Inhale through your nose and exhale through your mouth.

Again, inhale through your nose and this time as you exhale close your eyes.

Repeat this one more time and relax.

Sharpen your breathing focus.

Find stillness in every breath you take, relieve yourself from any tension and relax.

Let your body relax, soften your heart, quiet your anxious mind and open to whatever you experience without fighting.

Simply allow your thoughts and experiences to come and go without grasping at them.

Reduce any stress, anxiety, or negative emotions you might have, cool down become deeply and comfortably relaxed.

That's fine.

And as you continue to relax then you can begin the process of reprogramming your mind for your weight loss success because with the right mindset, then you can think positively about what you want to achieve. It begins with changing your mindset and attitude, because the key to losing weight all starts in the mind. One of the very first things you must throw out the window (figuratively) before you start your journey to weight loss is negativity. Negative thinking will just lead you nowhere. It will only pull your moods down which might trigger emotional eating. Thus, you'll eat more, adding up to that unwanted weight instead of losing it. Remember that you must need to break your old bad habits and one of them is negative self-talk. You need to change your negative mental views and turn them into positive ones. For example, instead of telling yourself after a few days of workout that nothing is happening or changing, tell yourself that you have done a set of physical activities you have never imagine you can or will do. Make it a point to pat yourself on the back for every little progress you make every day, may it be five additional crunches from what you did yesterday. Understand and accept that this process is a complete transformation, a metamorphosis if you will. This understanding is going to make the process smoother, and less painful.

Aside from being positive, you should also be realistic. Don't expect an immediate change in your body. Keep in mind that losing weight is not an overnight thing. It is a long-term process and gradual progress. Set and focus on your goals to keep that negativity at bay. Losing weight needs consistent reminders and focus on proper mental preparations. Always keep yourself motivated. Train yourself to think positive all the time.

Don't compare yourself to others, because it will not help you attain your goals in losing weight. First and foremost, keep in mind that each one of us has different body types and compositions. There is a certain diet that may work on you, but not so much for the others. Possibly, some people might need more carbohydrates in their diet, while you might need to drop that and add more protein in your meals. Each one of us is unique. Therefore, your diet plan will surely differ from the person next to you.

Comparing yourself to other people's progress is just a negative thought and will just be unhelpful to you. Remember, always keep a positive outlook and commit to it before you start your diet. For the sake of your long-term success, leave the comparison trap. You're not exactly like the people you idolize and they're not exactly like you and that's perfectly fine. Accept that, embrace that and move on with your personal goals.

Be realistic in setting your goals. Think about small and easy to achieve goals that will guide you towards a long term of healthy lifestyle changes. Your goals should be healthy for your body. If you want to truly lose weight and keep it off, it will be a slow uphill battle, with occasional dips and times you'll want to quit. If you expect progress too fast, you will eventually not be able to reach your goals and become discouraged. Don't add extra obstacles for yourself, plan your goals carefully.

If possible, try to find someone who has similar goals as you and work on them together. Two is always better than one, and having someone who understands what you are undergoing can be such a relief! An added benefit of having a partner-in-crime (or several) is that you can always hold each other accountable. Accountability is one thing that is easy to start being lax after the first few weeks of a new weight loss program, especially if results aren't quite where you want them to be.

Write down a realistic timetable that you can follow. Start a journal about your daily exercises and meal plan. You can cross out things that you have done already or add new ones along the way. Plot your physical activities. Make time and mark your calendar with daily physical activities. Try to incorporate at least a 15-minute workout on your busy days.

When you become aware of a thought or belief that pins the blame for your extra weight on something outside yourself, if you can find examples of people who've overcome that same cause, realize that it's decision time for you. Choose for yourself whether this is a thought you want to embrace and accept. Does this thought support you living your best life? Does it move you toward your goals, or does it give you an excuse not to go after them?

If you determine your thought no longer serves you, you get to choose another thought instead. Instead of pointing to some external, all-powerful cause for you being overweight, you can choose something different. Track your progress by writing down your step count or workouts daily to keep track of your progress.

Celebrate and embrace your results. Since the path to a healthy lifestyle is mostly hard work and discipline, try to reward yourself for every progress even if it is small. Treat yourself for a day of pampering, travel to a place you have been wanting to visit, go hiking, have a movie date with friends or get a new pair of shoes. These kinds of rewards provide you gratification and accomplishments that will make you keep going. Little things do count and little things also deserve recognition. But keep in mind that your rewards should not compromise your diet plan.

You can also do something like joining an athletic event, a fun run, where you can meet new people that share the same ideals of a healthy lifestyle. You get to learn more about weight loss from others and also share your knowledge. You need to find a source of motivation and keep that source of motivation fresh in your mind so you don't forget why you embarked on this journey to begin with.

As you focus on your journey of weight loss, keep your stress at bay because too much stress is harmful for the body in many ways, but it also can cause people to gain weight. When the body is under stress, the body will automatically release many hormones and among one of them is cortisol. When the body is under duress and stress, cortisol is released, is can ignite the metabolism, for a period of time. However, if the body remains in stressful conditions, the hormone cortisol will continue to be released, and actually slow down the metabolism resulting in weight gain.

Everyone experiences stress; there is just no getting around that fact. However, minimizing stressors, as well as learning how to manage the stress in your life will not only help you with you with losing weight, but it will also make a more attractive you! High stress in anyone's life often brings out the worst in people. When you are trying to get a man, you want them to see the best of you, not the stressed out you. While you are decreasing your stress level, you will want to increase the amount of sleep you get each night. Lack of sleep is a link to weight gain and because of this, ensuring adequate and appropriate sleep is crucial when trying to lose weight. Sleep is vital for the well-being of the body, and the ability for the mind to function, but it is also related to maintaining weight. If you are tired, make sure you sleep, rest or relax, so you are not prone to gaining weight. When a person gets more sleep, the hormone leptin will rise and when this happens the appetite decreases which will also decrease body weight.

Gratitude is important in this journey because it teaches you how to make peace with your body, no matter what shape, size or weight it has at the moment. It makes you look at your body with full acceptance and love, saying: "I'm grateful for my body the way it is." It stops you from beating yourself up for being overweight, unhealthy or out of shape. Be grateful for this learning experience, accept yourself the way you are, and take massive action to get your balance back.

When you express gratitude, you vibrate on a higher energy level, you are positive and happy, and you are simply in the state of satisfaction.

The more things you can find to be grateful for during your weight loss journey, the easier it will be to maintain a positive attitude and keep your motivation up.

It will also get you past those tough moments when you are feeling demotivated to take action and stick to the exercising or eating plan.

This means that you start expressing gratitude for the aspects of your body you would like to have, as if you already have them now. Be grateful for your sexy legs and slim waist. Be grateful for your increased energy levels and strength. Be grateful for the ability to wear smaller clothes. You get the drill. Feel the positive energy of gratitude flowing through your body as you imagine these things are true. By going through this exercise you'll notice the positive change in your thought patterns.

With the level of personal growth, you will achieve and the habits you will change on this session of hypnosis, you will feel like a completely different person. You will have more power, self–confidence and love yourself more than you ever thought possible before. That's change from the inside out. That's what lasts. And, at the end of the day, that's what truly matters.

Take a deep breath and allow your breath to return its natural rate as you return to your normal consciousness.

As you continue to breath, note that, right now, in this moment, you have no worries. You are just a relaxed body. Any distractions that arise while you tell yourself this can wait.

Repeat the following phrases:

- I am relaxed

- I am balanced
- I can deal with any worries later
- I am relaxed
- I am balanced

The whole earth supports you in your relaxation and balance. Feel yourself supported and held.

Feel that everything you have done in your life has brought you to this moment without errors or mistakes.

This moment is perfect.

Chapter 25:
The Psychology about Weight Loss

Weight Loss Is Hard

As you already know, weight loss is hard. It's intimidating, and often doesn't feel good. You put yourself through hell at the gym, and you start to dread having to get up and go through the same awful things that you think are necessary for losing weight. Losing weight becomes a burden rather than a satisfying process, and with this mindset, even if you manage to lose weight, you won't feel good about yourself in the way that you should when it's all over because you'll be swaddled by negative feelings.

During weight loss, your body will often fight against you and urge you to eat more even though that is against your diet plan. Hormonally and emotionally, you'll want to go back to eating how you used to. Hypnosis can help stave off the urges, but it helps to understand what you're up against because this information highlights that dieting takes a lot more than willpower to be successful. You need to gather all your weight loss tools, and you need to use them to undermine the hardships of weight loss, or else you'll never find the success that you want and deserve. Weight loss isn't impossible, but it can seem pretty grim, especially in the beginning when you're still getting your footing.

The statistics are not on your side. Very few people actually lose weight. Just over forty percent of men and fifty-six percent of women in the world tried to lose weight as of 2019. A whopping sixty percent of high school girls have tried to lose weight. Many people are trying to lose weight in the world at any given time, but an estimated eighty to ninety-five percent of people regain weight after losing it. Often, this regain is attributed to unmaintainable weight loss regimes that are often advertised. Weight loss can be straightforward, but keeping your weight down in the long term can be arduous. The contestants of "The Biggest Loser" show this. While some contestants of the notorious weight-loss show have been able to maintain their weight, most returned to their original weight within six years.

People often focus only on the weight loss element of physical transformation, but thinking about just weight loss itself isn't going to lead to actual results. If people refuse to acknowledge the psychological impacts of weight loss, our weight loss statistics will never improve. There's so much misinformation out there about weight loss, information that tells people they need to starve themselves and subscribe to extreme diets. People are being set up by failure by diets that promise fast results but give no emotional support or strategies for maintenance. Eating well for a while isn't going to cut the cravings. You have to change your mindset if you want to change your life.

They aren't making genuine, lasting changes to their lives. Even so, to succeed at weight loss, you need to take measures that other people don't. Hypnosis is one such step, and understanding why you might be reluctant to give your all to lifestyle changes is another important step you need to take. So many people are afraid of changes, which is why fear is one of the biggest mental blockers that you have to defeat before you can lose weight.

Don't Let Fears Hold You Back

Fears can be so damaging to your progress. It's almost impossible to commit yourself in the way you need to if you are so fixated on your fears instead of what you can do to succeed. Hypnosis is best done with willingness and openness, so don't let your fears hold you back and impede your ability to do what you've always wanted to do. Before you even start hypnosis, you need to analyze and understand what fears you have so that you can prepare for the major obstacles that will threaten your progress. Fears are valid; they stem from your brain wanting to protect you from danger, but you need to avoid overblowing them in your mind.

The fear of failure is one of the biggest fears that can disrupt your ability to give you all to losing weight. This fear can lead to you quit when you've only just gotten started. Nearly one-third of all adults in the United States have a fear of failure, and this fear can seep into every part of a person's life. It can make you feel insecure and unable to accomplish anything. This fear can make it hard to change anything too, and it can feel impossible to overcome the worry that you're just going to fail anyway. This fear can be draining because it makes you unhealthily obsessed with the things that could go wrong. Instead of thinking that you might succeed, you convince yourself that there's no chance that you will succeed. Then, you become a self-fulfilling prophecy and really do fail.

The fear of failure can easily lead to self-sabotage. When you fear failure, you'll avoid doing the things that could bring you success and choose the safety of stagnancy. You're not any happier by doing this, but psychologically, it feels safer. The truth is, though, that when you let your fears run your life, you're not better off because, in that scenario, you will never thrive. At least when taking a chance, you have the chance of triumph. When you have a fear of failure, you may subconsciously take measures to thwart your advancement. You will mess up, and then just quit because you feel like your progress has already been ruined.

You don't need to live with the fear of failure anymore. You can address this fear by knowing that you don't have to be perfect. You're human, and sometimes you're not going to do things in the best way. Hindsight allows you to see things that you didn't see before, and it can make you feel like a fool, but know that your mistakes don't mean you're a failure as a person. They are normal, and they are okay.

Look at your failures constructively. Don't even call them failures anymore because, more than anything, they are opportunities to grow. People often look at failure as something shameful, but when you have misfortune, it doesn't mean that you are incompetent or somehow bad. Use mistakes as a chance to grow. When you face failure, don't use that moment to give up or run away. Find ways you can improve. If you overeat one day, don't let yourself think that your whole diet is ruined because a good diet isn't shattered by one day of overindulgence. You need to understand that getting back on track is the biggest success you can have on this journey. For all the successes you have, you will have errors, but with a good outlook, those errors won't destroy you. They will build you up and help you learn through experience.

Imagine the worst that could happen if you put in a genuine effort. It's scary to think of the worst-case scenarios, but most of the time, the worst that you're thinking in your head is absurd and unlikely to happen. By letting yourself think of the worst that can happen, you can reduce the anxiety that you have regarding failure because the acknowledgment of what worries you is liberating. By identifying what is truly bothering you, you take away the power of that fear and can prepare yourself for any disappointment or negative feelings that you may face on your weight loss journey.

Take the pressure off yourself. Putting yourself under pressure isn't going to help you. It's just going to stress you out. Try not to put strict time parameters on your weight loss. Don't tell yourself, "I need to be ten pounds lighter by the holidays," because the pressure is going to get in your head and make it harder to stick to your diet. It's okay to want to accomplish certain goals by certain times, but if those goals don't happen at the exact time you want them too, you must avoid being hard on yourself. Sometimes, things happen, and you can no longer meet the expectations you had for yourself. That's fine, and you can adjust your expectations accordingly.

Find aspirations outside of weight loss that makes you happy so that you have other things to keep you going when you have mishaps. Your whole life shouldn't be single-mindedly focused on weight loss. If it is, you're probably miserable. You have to have other goals to strive for that have nothing to do with your weight. Find hobbies and activities that add excitement and happiness to your life because these will not only help you relax, but they will take your mind off food. It's hard to lose weight when you're thinking about food all the time, so let yourself think about other things. Be conscious about your dietary decisions, but don't allow weight to be the only thing that drives you.

The fear of not being enough or the fear of being an imposter are also fearing that many people deal with. Many people think that no matter what they do, they will never be good enough for all the good things that they have. These self-esteem issues make it hard to find the incentive and momentum to lose weight. The fear of not being enough often also feeds into imposter syndrome. Imposter syndrome is the fear people have that in certain areas of their lives, especially work, that they are imposters who seem to be competent at what they are doing to other people but are just pretending to have the necessary skills. They feel like imposters, faking their expertise to the people who they know, and they are terrified that they will be revealed as not being worthy of what they have. People with imposter syndrome are perfectly competent, but they feel as though everyone else will see them someday as being ineffectual, which can result in these people avoiding attention and trying not to make any major changes.

To make yourself feel worthy, you can do a myriad of things, but the most important thing is to find enjoyment in who you are. See beyond what your body looks like or how well you do your job. Tell yourself that you are worth it. Affirmations are a smart way to convince yourself that something is true. Your brain believes all the things that you tell it most; thus, by repeating positive things about yourself, you will build worth and start to value yourself as a person more.

Be unafraid to be yourself. Don't keep the things you love and want a secret. Feel free to share what you love, even if other people won't necessarily relate to those things. Sharing your passions is an ideal way to bond with the people around you, and when you share your passions, you're reiterating that you are worth it by allowing the things you love to be validated.

Chapter 26:
Women are Different from Men

The basic principles of weight loss are the same for both genders- you burn more calories than you consume- but the factors that lead to a caloric deficit that causes weight loss are not the same. Men and women are different. They are biologically different and emotionally different. These differences are very important because both biology and psychology are important for successful weight loss.

Different Bodies

There is no need to explain the physical differences between men and women. The body composition of men and women, that is, the proportions of muscle, bone, and fat that make up the body of men and women are very different. A typical 154-pound man has 69 pounds of muscle, 23 pounds of bone, and 23 pounds of fat (the rest is organs, fluids, etc.). A typical woman weighing 125 pounds weighs 45 pounds of muscle, 15 pounds of bone, and 34 pounds of fat. In summary, men are genetically programmed to have muscular build up with heavier bones than women. Conversely, the female body is designed for higher fat content.

Technically, the definitions of overweight and obesity are based upon the excess body fat (Body Mass Index or BMI is used to categorize the person's weight). Again, the gender is different. Obesity in men is defined as 21-25% body fat and obesity as 25% or more. Obesity in women is defined as 31-33% body fat and obesity as 33% or more. From a biological point of view, men should be lean in appearance, and women should be fat, so men and women of the same size and weight should have very different body compositions. Given the physical differences between sexes in terms of body composition, it is not surprising that body fat recommendations differ between men and women. Men are recommended a range of 12-20% fats, and women are recommended a range of 20-30%. Because of their different body composition, losing weight gives men a biological advantage over women.

Different Minds

Men and women do not share the same physical and psychological build-up. Differences based on emotions between men and women are a very interesting area. John Gray's 1992 book "Men are from Mars, Women are from Venus" attracted people's attention and sparked a debate on the inherent differences between men and women in communication, addressing problems, and causing conflict. Psychologists are not the only ones interested in how mental processes differ between women and men. Much work is also done in the world of basic research. Every year, more and more are learned about the relationship between mental processes and physical functioning, especially concerning neurotransmitters. A 2006 article even states that men smile less than women, were due to how their brains were programmed. It is well known that chemical behaviors in the brain influence our behaviors in the areas of food and physical activity. Also, although little is known about these signals at this time, there may be differences due to gender. The brain is associated with the potential effects of obesity and gender, so the more we learn about how the brain affects mental health, the more relevant treatment options will be developed. The mental aspect of weight and weight loss cannot be overemphasized. The basic physiology of weight loss is relatively simple. To lose weight, you need to lose more and ingest fewer calories. One needs to know that at the heart of permanent weight loss is the behavior of eating, exercising, and thinking. There is a clear difference between men and women when it comes to weight loss.

Health Risk Obesity for Women

Women and men share the health risks of certain diseases, but some weight-related health problems are found only in women. Weight loss seems to be one of the most important ways for women to overcome these problems beyond the potential health risks. Example:

Polycystic Ovary Syndrome (PCOS) is a condition that can affect a woman's fertility and is associated with obesity. Health professionals recommend weight loss as the first treatment for PCOS because studies have shown that losing weight improves fertility.

Besides, obesity is a risk factor for Gestational Diabetes. Studies show that a weight loss of just 10 pounds can significantly reduce a woman's risk of developing gestational diabetes.

Adult obesity and weight gain are also known risk factors for Postmenopausal Breast Cancer. In an analysis of a large group of women in Iowa, researchers found that preventing weight gain at childbearing age, or preventing weight gain in overweight women combined with weight loss, was healthy during those years. It was concluded that maintaining a healthy weight reduced the risk of being diagnosed with breast cancer in later years.

Overweight negatively affect the psychological health of both genders but appears to be more emotionally stressful for women (Emotional Stress). Studies show that women are less satisfied with weight and overall body shape than men. And most women's dissatisfaction with weight begins early in life and continues into adulthood. Why? The answer lies, at least partially, in an attachment to the lean body for women in almost all societies.

Weight watcher researchers often hear women say they feel that others are judging them by their appearance (thin and attractive), not by what they are capable of and what they can do. Where do women get this belief? The media is an important source of information. Most of the beautiful women in magazines and big screens are extraordinarily thin people, and for many women, extraordinary thinness is a measure of beauty. This seems to be primarily a woman's problem.

A study that asked men and women for their ideal body shape and asked how they thought of their body in comparison with their ideals was generally satisfied. In contrast, women consistently viewed themselves as heavier than their ideals and expressed a desire to lose weight. Unfortunately, this very thin waif character is unrealistic (and unhealthy!) And can't be achieved by most women. As a result, many women lose self-esteem and develop a negative body image associated with depression.

So, instead of focusing on being extremely thin, one should focus on maintaining a healthy weight. Now, we will finally move to actual weight loss techniques for losing extra fats. We will be focusing on the root of the problem, the brain.

Chapter 27:
Blasting Calories

We have all heard the word "calorie" and its relation to our body weight. Calories are contained in the foods we consume and are often misunderstood about how they affect us. In this topic, we seek to explain what they are, how to count them, and the best methods of blasting them to avoid weight gain.

What are Calories, and how do they affect Your Weight?

A calorie is a key estimating unit. For example, we use meters when communicating separation;' Usain Bolt went 100 meters in simply 9.5 seconds.' There are two units in this expression. One is a meter (a range unit), and the other is "second" (a period unit). Essentially, calories are additional units of physical amount estimation.

Many assume that a calorie is the weight measure (since it is oftentimes connected with an individual's weight). That is not precise, however. A calorie is a vitality unit (estimation). 1 calorie is proportional to the vitality expected to build the temperature by 1 degree Celsius to 1 kilogram of water.

Two particular sorts of calories come in: small calories and huge calories. Huge calories are the word connected to sustenance items.

You've likely observed much stuff on parcels (chocolates, potato chips, and so forth.) with' calorie scores.' Imagine the calorie score an incentive for a thing being' 100 cal.' this infers when you eat it, you will pick up about as much vitality (even though the calorie worth expressed and the amount you advantage from it is never the equivalent).

All that we eat has a particular calorie tally; it is the proportion of the vitality we eat in the substance bonds.

These are mostly things we eat: starches, proteins, and fats. How about we take a gander at what number of calories 1 gram comprises of these medications: 1. Sugars 4 calories 2. Protein–3 calories. Fat–nine calories

Are my calories awful?

That is fundamentally equivalent to mentioning, "Is vitality awful for me?" Every single activity the body completes needs vitality. Everything takes vitality to stand, walk, run, sit, and even eat. In case you're doing any of these tasks, it suggests you're utilizing vitality, which mostly infers you're' consuming' calories, explicitly the calories that entered your body when you were eating some nourishment.

To sum things up, for you, NO... calories are not terrible.

Equalization is the way to finding harmony between what number of calories you devour and what number of calories you consume or use. On the off chance that you eat fewer calories and spend more, you will become dainty, while on the opposite side, on the off chance that you gobble up heaps of calories, however, you are a habitually lazy person, you will in the long run become stout at last.

Each movement we do throughout a day will bring about certain calories being spent. Here is a little rundown of the absolute most much of the time performed exercises, just as the number of calories consumed while doing them.

Step by step instructions to Count Calories

You have to expend fewer calories than you consume to get thinner.

This clamor is simple in principle. Be that as it may, it very well may be hard to deal with your nourishment admission in the contemporary sustenance setting. Calorie checking is one approach to address this issue and is much of the time used to get more fit. Hearing that calories don't make a difference is very common, and tallying calories is an exercise in futility. Nonetheless, calories tally with regards to your weight; this is a reality that, in science, analyses called overloading studies has been demonstrated on numerous occasions.

These examinations request that people deliberately indulge and after that, survey the impact on their weight and wellbeing. All overloading investigations have found that people are putting on weight when they devour a bigger number of calories than they consume.

This simple reality infers that calorie checking and limiting your utilization can be proficient in averting weight put on or weight reduction as long as you can stick to it. One examination found that health improvement plans, including calorie including brought about a normal weight reduction of around 7 lbs. (3.3 kg) more than those that didn't.

Primary concern: You put on weight by eating a larger number of calories than you consume. Calorie tallying can help you expend fewer calories and get more fit.

How many calories do you have to eat?

What number of calories you need depends on factors, for example, sex, age, weight, and measure of activity? For example, a 25-year-old male competitor will require a bigger number of calories than a non-practicing 70-year-elderly person. In case you're endeavoring to get in shape, by eating not exactly your body consumes off, you'll have to construct a calorie deficiency. Utilize this adding machine to decide what number of calories you ought to expend every day (opening in crisp tab). This number cruncher depends on the condition of Mifflin-St Jeor, an exact method to evaluate calorie prerequisites.

How to Reduce your Caloric Intake for Weight Loss

Bit sizes have risen, and a solitary dinner may give twofold or triple what the normal individual needs in a sitting at certain cafés. "Segment mutilation" is the term used to depict enormous parts of sustenance as the standard. It might bring about weight put on and weight reduction. In general, people don't evaluate the amount they spend. Tallying calories can help you battle indulging by giving you a more grounded information of the amount you expend.

In any case, you have to record portions of sustenance appropriately for it to work. Here are a couple of well-known strategies for estimating segment sizes: Scales: Weighing your sustenance is the most exact approach to decide the amount you eat. This might be tedious, in any case, and isn't constantly down to earth.

Estimating cups: Standard estimations of amount are, to some degree, quicker and less complex to use than a scale, yet can some of the time be tedious and unbalanced.

Examinations: It's quick and easy to utilize correlations with well-known items, especially in case you're away from home. It's considerably less exact, however.

Contrasted with family unit items, here are some mainstream serving sizes that can help you gauge your serving sizes: 1 serving of rice or pasta (1/2 a cup): a PC mouse or adjusted bunch.

- 1 Meat serving (3 oz): a card deck.
- 1 Fish serving (3 oz): visit book.
- 1 Cheese serving (1.5 oz): a lipstick or thumb size.
- 1 Fresh organic product serving (1/2 cup): a tennis ball.
- 1 Green verdant vegetable serving (1 cup): baseball.
- 1 Vegetable serving (1/2 cup): a mouse PC.

- 1 Olive oil teaspoon: 1 fingertip.
- 2 Peanut margarine tablespoons: a ping pong ball.

Calorie tallying, notwithstanding when gauging and estimating partitions, isn't a careful science.

In any case, your estimations shouldn't be thoroughly spot-on. Simply guarantee that your utilization is recorded as effectively as would be prudent. You ought to be mindful to record high-fat as well as sugar things, for example, pizza, dessert, and oils. Under-recording these meals can make an enormous qualification between your genuine and recorded utilization. You can endeavor to utilize scales toward the begin to give you a superior idea of what a segment resembles to upgrade your evaluations. This should help you to be increasingly exact, even after you quit utilizing them.

More Tips to Assist in Caloric Control

Here are 5 more calorie tallying tips:

- Get prepared: get a calorie tallying application or web device before you start, choose how to evaluate or gauge parcels, and make a feast plan.
- Read nourishment marks: Food names contain numerous accommodating calorie tallying information. Check the recommended segment size on the bundle.
- Remove the allurement: dispose of your home's low-quality nourishment. This will help you select more advantageous bites and make hitting your objectives easier.

- Aim for moderate, steady loss of weight: don't cut too little calories. Even though you will get in shape all the more rapidly, you may feel terrible and be less inclined to adhere to your arrangement.

- Fuel your activity: Diet and exercise are the best health improvement plans. Ensure you devour enough to rehearse your vitality.

Effective Methods for Blasting Calories

To impact calories requires participating in exercises that urge the body to utilize vitality. Aside from checking the calories and guaranteeing you eat the required sum, consuming them is similarly basic for weight reduction. Here, we examine a couple of techniques that can enable you to impact our calories all the more viably.:

1) Indoor cycling: McCall states that around 952 calories for each hour ought to be at 200 watts or higher. On the off chance that the stationary bicycle doesn't demonstrate watts: "This infers you're doing it when your indoor cycling instructor educates you to switch the opposition up!" he proposes.

2) Skiing: around 850 calories for every hour depends on your skiing knowledge. Slow, light exertion won't consume nearly the same number of calories as a lively, fiery exertion is going to consume. To challenge yourself and to consume vitality? Attempt to ski tough.

3) Rowing: Approximately 816 calories for every hour. The benchmark here is 200 watts; McCall claims it ought to be at a "fiery endeavor." Many paddling machines list the showcase watts. Reward: Rowing is additionally a stunning back exercise.

4) Jumping rope: About 802 calories for each hour This ought to be at a moderate pace—around 100 skips for each moment—says McCall. Attempt to begin with this bounce rope interim exercise.

5) Kickboxing: Approximately 700 calories for every hour. Also, in this class are different sorts of hand to hand fighting, for example, Muay Thai. With regards to standard boxing, when you are genuine in the ring (a.k.a. battling another individual), the biggest calorie consumption develops. Be that as it may, many boxing courses additionally incorporate cardio activities, for example, hikers and burpees, so your pulse will in the long run increment more than you would anticipate. What's more, hello, before you can get into the ring, you need to start someplace, isn't that so?

6) Swimming: Approximately 680 calories for each hour Freestyle works, however as McCall says, you should go for a vivacious 75 yards for each moment. For an easygoing swimmer, this is somewhat forceful. (Butterfly stroke is significantly progressively productive if you extravagant it.)

7) Outdoor bicycling: Approximately 680 calories for each hour biking at a fast, lively pace will raise your pulse, regardless of whether you are outside or inside. Add to some rocky landscape and mountains and gets significantly more calorie consuming.

The volume of calories devoured is straightforwardly proportionate to the measure of sustenance, just like the kind of nourishment an individual expends. The best way to lessen calories is by being cautious about what you devour and captivating in dynamic physical exercises to consume overabundance calories in your body.

Chapter 28:
Great Techniques to Reach Your Ideal Weight

1. You jot down each move when you go through the techniques, is essential. Get a pen and paper, and let's work through the techniques step by step.

2. Have you ever tried weight loss in the past? Did you succeed? That was the product of your preceding attempt to lose weight, now try to define what you've done. If you haven't been successful, be frank with yourself and list the reasons that contributed to your failure.

3. Identify the future weight loss plan's strengths, shortcomings, incentives and risks. Twenty per cent of your muscles will spur you on to your target weight, following the ideals of the 80/20 rules.

4. Set the expectations. Be sure how you plan to make your ideal weight come true. Your targets must be clear, observable, achievable, practical and time bound. Here's the contrast between what a good is and perhaps a wrong goal.

5. Write a plan of action for how you'll accomplish your goal — word of caution here. You need to get your action plan written down. You'll be failing without writing down your course of action.

   Plan of action: o Weigh myself and record weight in my diary before I launch my program for rapid weight loss.

- Weigh myself at 7 pm every Monday and record how much I weigh in the diary.
- Walk at least 1 mile in the neighborhood every evening between 5 pm and 6 pm.
- Drink 10 cups of water (100 MLS per glass) a day.
- Eat breakfast high in fiber content any day of the week.
- Listen to hypnotic audio message weight loss before I get off to bed.

6. Implement the Course of Action. Act, and do the acts. You have to act, or you're never going to achieve your goal.

7. Read your written target and the action plan each morning when you wake, and then you go to bed in the evening. This will get you working on your plans. Create copies of the target and plan of action and put them all over the house to always remind you.

8. Take a look at your growth. Concentrate on your strengths, persevere and remain consistent.

9. Visualize yourself to have weight loss.

10. Let's be optimistic. Never doubt your efforts to lose weight. Never seek to focus on your shortcomings.

11. Be bold in incorporating many weight-loss strategies in the action plan, like hypnosis and some others.

The Risk of Rapid Weight Loss. Most individuals who would like to lose weight wants to make it happen as soon as possible. After all the same thing that helps us gain weight just does it due to eating pleasure. And weight loss is viewed as painful.

And the more quickly you can shed the extra weight, the better, right?

Incorrect. Quick weight loss is only one long-term failure recipe. If you have a strict low-calorie diet, or if you have prolonged fasting, your body feels it is in danger. People led a life of festivity or famine in the earliest days of hunter-gatherers.

Typically the body would go into a frustrating process in times of drought, holding on to fat until it could find another source of food.

An extreme diet will lead to weight loss since your body will begin to use fat reserves only after your food reserves are burned up. But that's going to slow this process fast.

The rapid weight loss is not only a fat loss. There is a lot of depletion of the gas. You get hydrated beneath and your body changes even more. Dehydration generates significant health issues. Another major problem is the lack of muscle.

Muscle failure is challenging to recover from. Building only one kilo of muscle needs lots of exercises. But if you do a drastic weight-loss plan, you will lose it quickly.

When you start a deficient calorie diet, one example would be to lose 4 kilograms in a week. It may be two kilograms of fat, one kilogram of muscle and one kilogram of air. You think this diet can't be managed, so you quit. You've put the four kilos back on within a few weeks.

But most likely it will be one kilo of oil and three kilograms of fat due to it's easy to put on fat ante tryout to put on muscle. You are now back at your old weight. And you've got more fat and less muscle. That means you'll have less capacity to burn fat.

You will lose some muscle with every subsequent weight-loss effort.

The secret to proper weight loss is to gradually and sustainably lose weight. Your body can comfortably cope with just half a kilo per week. Plus you'll preserve your muscle mass if you do routine exercise. Additionally, make sure that you are adequately hydrated. This offers you the most excellent chance to achieve your perfect weight and hold it.

Over the years, due to stage hypnotists as well as media, how hypnosis can help you lose weight Hypnosis has earned a bad reputation. It is time to change this as hypnosis is a compelling technique if you want to alter any aspect of your personality. Knowing how to use hypnosis is the perfect way of preventing the use of it. If you've tried hypnosis of weight loss but refused to use this approach because of anxiety, don't let it deter you any longer. All that you heard about hypnosis is nothing but myths.

Most of these people would love to be smaller, but none would like to do some job. Typically these are people who have tried a lot of diets, and they can't lose weight or lose the weight they want for any reason.

Hypnosis is an advantageous method which helps people like you quickly and easily lose weight. Hypnosis is often associated with stigma due to confusion and misconceptions, but hypnosis is a hugely successful method of helping with weight loss.

Weight gain is mostly attributed to overeating and lack of physical activity. The issue is, the signs of the problem are these and not the cause. The cause is concealed underneath the surface, and virtually every diet only discusses the symptoms of the surface rather than the actual cause.

Emotional or behavioral problems typically caused unnecessary eating and lack of weight gain – causing activity. That may be an urge to hide from the world and not be heard, so you're gaining weight. It could be an urge in the past to punish yourself for any actual sin or imagine it. This might be almost anything, so it's going to be a source of emotional or emotion.

Although you can lose the weight by dieting and through your exercise, it would be difficult to hold the weight off unless you also tackle the psychological issues that caused the weight loss initially.

The first misconception concerning hypnosis is that the methods are all alike. There could not be anything further from the facts. Authoritarian hypnosis, "You get sleepy", is the one that most people think about when they hear about this process. Very few people work with this kind. They are looking for a doctor who uses such approaches as clinical counselling and communication while you're attempting weight loss hypnosis. The oppressive hypnotist also scares away people by dictating what they will do. The behavioral hypnotizer, on the other hand, works for you. He is trying to understand better you're eating habits and how it affects your weight issue. The keys to this approach are motivation and positive reinforcement.

Hypnosis misconception number two centers around the subliminal messages. Subliminal messages are those you don't listen to. Among other stuff, they're potentially found in ads that you use. There has been a lot of discussion about this sort of post. In reality, at one point, people assumed that LP records contained subliminal messages and they were afraid that many musicians would be listening to children. The subliminal messages do not work if you care and think about it. Only because you hear anything doesn't mean that you can act on it. Work is carrying this out. Subliminal messages aren't working.

The third myth relating to hypnosis is widespread. Many people think no tool will hypnotize them. This approach will support an incredibly large portion of the population. It is known that it is not possible to captivate even those with deficient intelligence or those with brain damage. Whether or not you can be hypnotized is more a hypnotist factor, not your hypnotizing capacity. To be successful, a hypnotist must be versatile.

Myth number four of hypnosis is that this is a weird practice that you encourage everyone to do to your brain and body. In reality, hypnosis is nothing more than using your normal dream state, the one often refers to as REM (rapid eye movement), intentionally. Sleep is a form of hypnosis you commit to every day. Hypnosis of weight loss works since it's normal.

The fifth myth relating to hypnosis is that during the process, you lose control of both the mind and body. We've all seen television shows depicting a person clucking like a chicken while being hypnotized. Real hypnosis is nothing more than a calming condition where you are intensely concentrated. By trying to take your attention away from the specialist, you may stop the process at any time. It could not be any simpler.

It is here that hypnosis comes into its own. Hypnosis helps to dig into the subconscious mind and address the problems that cause the increase of weight.

Hypnosis aid can be accessed in two ways.

Next, you should see a clinical hypnotist and also have one session on one. These are very successful but can be a little costly. You need to make sure that you locate a suitably trained and competent hypnotist. You won't usually need more than 5-8 sessions to lose weight permanently. If a hypnotist tells you to need more than that, then shop around a little bit more. The easiest way to find a successful clinical hypnotist is to give a personal recommendation.

The most rapid effect is provided by using both vocal and subliminal. The spoken form leads you through a session of hypnosis, which is best listened to when you will not be disturbed. The subliminal variant can usually be heard everywhere, as long as there are no binaural beats in it. When it has binaural beats, then relaxing ramps up and should not be heard when driving or running machinery.

All the rage among today's Hollywood stars is hypnosis for weight loss, and rightly so. Not only are they drop-dead magnificent and ideally physically fit to see spectacular and rapid results using this form, but by getting into the Hollywood secret on average every day, Joes like you and I lose pounds and inches quickly.

In a psychological research evaluation, it has been found that over 90% of participants who engaged in weight loss hypnosis trials lost significantly more weight than those who did not undergo any form of hypnotic therapy. The numbers speak for themselves, very quietly.

Conclusion

Most people claim that weight loss hypnosis is a simple way to solve weight issues. People are also attracted by hypnosis because they feel they don't have to do any workouts, they can eat whatever they want, and all they have to do is close their eyes and lose weight in minutes. That's just not true.

No magic pills are available to lose weight, be it by hypnosis or some other form of weight loss. It is not possible to lose weight immediately after only one hypnosis session. A well-trained and professional hypnotist takes many sessions to achieve the best possible outcomes.

Several websites on the Internet say that weight loss hypnosis will produce dramatic results after just one session. Most people are likely to be insulted by this argument because everybody knows it is not possible to lose the weight overnight-however successful the hypnotist is.

Practicing weight loss hypnosis was another method for those who want to shape their bodies as they wish. There are also men who don't like their own body image. This leads to loss of self-esteem and confidence. Some people prefer to use workouts and other lifestyle strategies to achieve their ideal body shape. Unfortunately, few tests are churning out. That is why people who understood the technique of mental strength resort to hypnosis to lose their body mass. You will find an absolute guide on how to use that method to attain the correct body shape on the internet. It is up to you to use your brain's strength to understand how useful it can be for you.

Hypnotizing is generally known to remove the inner self concentration. It generally happens in the same way as in a trance. Slimming hypnosis is an operation performed with the aid of the hypnotherapist. In this case, the person who wants to slightly repeat the messages given to him in the form of sentences, phrases, or even pictures may do so verbally. Mental images often play a major role in achieving the same result.

One thing you must remember is that your mind needs to concentrate more as you go through the hypnotizing process. In certain states, the mind and the subconscious state are very sensitive. You are well-positioned to react suggestively to the circumstances which lead you to your ideal body so that the best results can be obtained in a very short period of time. It is an activity that many people can do effectively with much less effort.

The research centers and interested stakeholders have performed many studies. Research has shown that people typically achieve fair outcomes using this form of hypnosis. This method can also lose up to an average of 2.7 kilograms.

Hypnotized, however, does not always function well on its own. You will take into account other behaviors that can effectively improve your weight loss. Take the best diet plan with your nutritionist's support. Not just this, you should do the workouts that will reduce your excess weight. In addition, you will try to follow a balanced lifestyle, which would help you in the end. Regulate your sleep hours, for example, and avoid any bad habits.

If you use this routine and use all the tricks, you get the best performance. Ultimately, you learn to regulate your mind to lose weight. You train your subconscious mind to decrease your body mass, and if you practice this cycle, it will happen.

CPSIA information can be obtained
at www.ICGtesting.com
Printed in the USA
LVHW021649141120
671495LV00001B/69